INSOMNIUM

Insomnium

JOHN O'NEILL

Indy Pub

*To my grandpa, who gave me both his
name, and his love of learning.*

Prologue

You lie awake in your bedroom, staring at the ceiling. You want to get up and run away, but you cannot move. A panic, buzzing like a current of electricity, runs through every cell in your body. What caused it? Will you ever stop feeling this way? Is this what someone feels like when they lose their sanity? You do not know, and it does not matter. All that matters to you now is that your arms and legs feel like they have never moved before, your stomach is on fire, and your chest feels as though it might implode any moment.

The ceiling is dark and featureless. All of the details of your surroundings fade behind the white noise of your own terrified thoughts. Your questions zig-zag through your head. You reconsider every mistake that you have made throughout your life. You debate whether or not you deserve any of the good that has come to you. You fear the suffering that awaits you in the future. You try to breathe deeply but it does not help. Your lungs feel two sizes too small.

You want to get in a car and drive. You would press down on the gas pedal until every last drop of fuel is used up and the car would not move an inch further. And then you would get out of the car and start to run. Until you might reach somewhere beautiful, or at least somewhere far away from this moment. All of these things you would do if you were not so damn scared.

Of the consequences. Of hurting the people you care about. And most of all, of the unknown.

Just as you return to the question of if this miserable feeling will ever end, a pale glow appears in your doorway. Your more abstract, existential fears give way to very real ones. You think only of survival now and brace yourself for anything. You remember the baseball bat stowed just beneath your bed.

Then you hear a voice. It is calm, soothing, and feminine.

"Be still," the voice suggests. "I do not seek to harm you. In fact, I believe I may be able to help you."

You gradually raise your eyes to look at the source of these words. The woman is blindingly bright, especially to eyes that have spent several hours adjusting to the darkness of this bedroom. Faintly, some details can be seen. She has golden skin and wears a flowing gown with a veil over her head. This is all you can take in before the pain in your eyes forces you to look away. Even with your hand shielding your face you can tell that she is advancing. The glow is getting brighter.

"I have felt your suffering and wish to guide you towards healing. The process will not be easy, but I believe that it is necessary."

As she finishes her sentence she arrives at the edge of the bed. She glows to the point that the whole room appears to be bathed in sunlight. In your fear of this intruder you scramble to the far side of the mattress. With all of the courage in your body you manage to croak out, "Who are you?"

The woman seems to smile then, and somehow the glow becomes even stronger. Is each of her teeth a small sun?

"Do you see? There! There is some bravery within you. You will need it for the road ahead."

You feel her touch your hand, and you jump back. You sit now as far from her as you can get while still remaining on your bed. Though desperate to keep a watchful eye on her, you can still not look at the intruder directly. Instead you cover your eyes with your hands.

"Take my hand and I will lead you to the beginning."

Between your fingers you can see her hand extend towards you. Every motion you have seen her make since appearing has been elegant and slow.

But you cannot take her hand. This must be some elaborate plan to kidnap you. Perhaps when you lower your guard, she will produce whatever weapon she is hiding under her gown. Maybe she is simply distracting you while her associates steal everything you own in the other room.

You prepare to lunge at her and defend yourself with every ounce of courage you have. You make a fist and cock back your arm, just like a superhero would do. You finally look at her face to find a target for this punch, and in doing so you meet her gaze for the first time. Her eyes are like nothing you have ever seen before. They are purple, with no black dot in the middle for the pupil. Immediately you are hypnotized. Your fist relaxes, and your hand begins to reach out for hers. You do not stop it. Somehow, all of this makes sense. You are where you need to be, and you are doing what you need to be doing.

As your fingers touch you are swallowed by the bright light that surrounds your visitor. The light overpowers you, and you are forced to close your eyes.

Mountainside

You are on a mountain, confused about how you wound up here. Your first sensation is the wind nearly blowing you off your feet. You can tell by its force that you are very high up. You can tell by its temperature that you would no longer like to be here.

The wind applies a subtly changing pressure to the sides of your face and torso. It swirls around you and tousles your hair. You breathe in a portion of the air it provides, and the shock of cold air hitting your lungs wakes you up, and makes you feel more aware.

You scan your surroundings. The ominous entrance to a cave lies in front of you. It is a hole in the dark stone that covers the sides of this mountain. The opening itself is pure black and provides no further information about what the cave may hold. Choosing to avoid the uncertainty that you are sure that route would provide, you turn to find your way back down the path that you assume is behind you. After all, you had to get up here somehow.

But there is no path. Instead, you find a sheer drop-off that appears to stretch down to depths that would cause the Mariana Trench to feel inadequate. You see that you stand on a stone platform about twenty feet wide and ten feet long. It is the lone island of horizontal ground that you can see on the mountain's side.

Stretching out in front of you, there appears to be perfect nothingness. A dull fog obscures any sense of night or day. The ether swirls and undulates, giving the impression that it could be masking a silent war between giants, or nothing at all. You can see most of your mountain environment, though no other surrounding landforms, nor any way to travel up or down its sides.

Suddenly, you remember the strange Glowing Woman. Where is she?

"Hello!", you call out.

You hear no response, only the echoes of your own voice. Useless.

Have you been drugged? Did the woman and her henchmen carry you up to this mountain and leave you to die? If so, how did they escape? Were you dropped from a helicopter? No, you decide. You cannot hear the sound of any engines in the distance. It is completely silent here. They could not have climbed either, as mountain is far too steep and smooth.

You turn back to the cave. Its dark secrets are your only remaining option. You now notice the ribbons of lava, colored black now that they have hardened, carelessly adorning the rock all around the mouth of the cave. They paint this wall as an artist might, if the artist was drunk to the point of forgetting their own name. The ribbons present a picture of the birth of this mountain; of how it has grown and changed over its many years of existence.

Your focus returns to the path ahead of you. The entrance to the cave still appears to be a wall of black that your eyes cannot penetrate. While staring deep into its depths, contemplating your decision, you think you see some amount of movement. The prospect of finding some creature ahead requires another several minutes of mental preparation.

Eventually you become certain of the situation. You have been left up here to die, and your captors believe that you are incapable of surviving. The Glowing Woman's words ring through your mind.

There is some bravery within you! You will need it for the road ahead.

The sentiment sounds mocking now. She saw no bravery, just a coward that could be taken advantage of.

But, why? You may never know.

And so, two options remain. You can stay here and die, proving those villains right, or you can move forward and prove them wrong. Or at least attempt to. The road before you seems terrifying, but it provides a chance at survival. At least it can be written on your tombstone that you took the path of hope. Without any other options, you take a deep breath, steel yourself for whatever horrors await you, and plunge into the darkness.

The cave envelops you quickly, and within a few steps you cannot tell the difference between your eyes being open or closed. You lose sight of the entrance to the cave soon, its light fading behind one of the many bends in the tunnel. You run your hand along the wall beside you and take each step slowly and deliberately. The floor is firm and smooth. You soon grow confident that each new step will provide no surprises. The wall is damp and cool to the touch. Its slightly jagged texture is interrupted only by occasional patches of moss. This harmless vegetation causes you to jump in fear of having woken up one of the many poisonous spiders that would presumably live in such a creepy place.

The cave begins to take not only your sense of sight but of time as well. Your blind walk feels as though it continues for hours, though with some focused thought you realize it has most likely only been a few minutes. Uncertainty weighs heavily on your mind, and you begin to rethink your strategy.

Just as you begin to consider returning to the dull light of the cliff, you sense that you are no longer walking through darkness. At some point, you had apparently given up on your eyes entirely and closed them, unconsciously choosing to trust your other senses. Now your eyelids mask what appears to be a bright glow all around you. Cautiously, you allow them to part.

Valley

You blink your eyes as they adjust to the light that now surrounds you. Your new environment gradually comes into view. Before you lies a vast green expanse, with a few trees dotting an otherwise unobstructed grassy field. Two walls of stone rise up at either side of this valley, hundreds of feet apart, and extend up into a thick layer of clouds. You cannot see the top of these cliffs. You suppose that you have walked straight through the tunnel and are now on the other side of the mountain that you began on. Out of curiosity, you turn around to see how far you meandered before realizing that you had left the tunnel. To your surprise, you find only more grass behind you. There is no sign of the cave nor its tunnel. It is almost as if you were dropped in the middle of this field, yet you distinctly remember walking in order to arrive here. Your concerns about insanity return full force.

Feeling very exposed out in the open like this, you walk towards one of the great walls of stone that frame this pasture. In the distance you can see a stream running through the valley. You decide that it might be wise to make your way there instead, to find what you hope to be clean water. After all, being lost on a mysterious mountain can be exhausting, and you should take any chance at sustenance that you get.

As you move through the valley, you become aware of the weather. The clouds overhead are dark and foreboding. The wind is swirling and constantly changing, which appears to be giving the trees a difficult time of deciding in which direction to sway. There is an aroma in the air that can only be found when a storm is near. It is as though the air has suddenly condensed and you can feel the water hanging within it. While the prospect of rain sounds fairly refreshing to you, your pleasant mood shifts to concern when you remember how exposed you are in this open field. You could very easily be struck by lightning in circumstances like this. This appears to be the first true threat to your surviving this ordeal. You cannot risk anything. You must confront the Glowing Woman. You attempt to stay close to the few trees scattered along your path.

Slowly but surely you make your way to the stream, walking about a mile to arrive there. From a closer view you can see that it is not particularly wide, only opening up ten feet at a maximum. As you reach its edge you can see that it is fairly deep. Its bottom is lined with rocks that glisten despite the sky's darkness. The water seems oddly stagnant for a stream of this size. In the reflection you see a familiar glow.

"Wouldn't it feel nice to unclog this river, and let it flow freely?"

You spin around to face the Glowing Woman again. She seems less radiant than before, allowing you to finally get a good look at her. Your supposed kidnapper is tall and thin, with pale golden skin and dark hair. Her eyes, though still bright purple, have a kind of warm, welcome feeling to them. She smiles gently at you from beneath her golden veil.

"Why am I here? Where even are we?" You ask the obvious questions first.

She smirks at these, and replies cryptically: "On some level you wish to be here, and I have not taken you far."

Before you can interrogate her further, she leaps into the water, and disappears as a flash of light racing downstream.

Great, you think, not only have you been left for dead in a strange place, but your captor seems to be magic.

She did raise a good point, though. Maybe there is some sort of man-made dam nearby that is causing the water to flow so slowly. Maybe there you can find some help. With a plan of action in your head, you set off upstream.

The storm above is holding off for the time being, but still lingers above. You almost wish it would just get on with it. The stream bends and twists its way along, doing its very best to follow the contours of the valley that it lies within. It appears to support no life, apart from the algae collecting in the stagnant water.

Despite this the water remains fairly clear, suggesting that it might not have been blocked for very long.

For a while it seems as though you will not find any blockage. The river stretches on and on with no dam in sight. Disappointed by this, you choose to admire the landscape to pass the time. The weather still seems volatile, and you are beginning to feel the occasional droplet of water fall from the sky.

The entire valley is lush and green. The soil, though red and seemingly belonging in a desert, is damp, keeping the imprint of your foot long after you have passed by. The clouds above swirl in the breeze. Thick, foggy tendrils hang down and curl around the higher parts of great rock walls at either side of the valley.

The walls themselves have bands of vegetation growing along their faces, persevering against the pull of gravity. The rock making up the walls is reddish in hue but varies in its darkness. It lends the behemoths a striped pattern. You remark to yourself that horizontal stripes often make a person appear thinner, and wonder if the rocks knew this when they got dressed. It becomes clear to you now that the soil beneath your feet eroded from the sides of the canyon, as they share the same color.

There are patches of shrubs growing on the banks of the stream, hiding its distinct edges with their leaves. As you attempt to look through the brush, you hear a soft gurgling and notice a pile of stones and sticks. It appears you have found the block in the river.

This natural dam, though not perfect, is succeeding in stopping the majority of the flow in the river. Behind the dam, a steady current charges forward with purpose. In front of it, a trickle of water flows at a speed that would be outdone by the average kitchen faucet. You look all around the little dam and see no signs of life. Inspecting the structure more carefully, it does not appear to be the work of human hands. You can see that it is made of rocks and twigs rather than bricks or cement. But the flow of water just seems so pathetic as you look down at it. With no other plan of action, you decide to wade in and remove the blockage while you plan your next move.

The riverbed is soft and sandy on your feet. The water, though stagnant and a bit murky, is cool and refreshing. You take a few moments to enjoy the sensation. Without any current, the water idles about your legs and does not prevent you from walking. This task becomes more difficult as the coldness of the water causes your toes to go slightly numb. Still, the water feels refreshing. The experience of stepping in at first feels as though your legs were bathed in mint leaves, and the tingling sensation does not fade for some time.

With your appreciation of the stream complete, you set to work on clearing the dam. In moving the various twigs and stones, you realize how the structure accomplished its task. While the rocks and branches are the main obstructions, the true cause of the blockage is the moss and weeds that are caught on them. As they flowed down the stream, they appear to have wedged themselves in the cracks between the rocks or wrap themselves around the sticks. In this way, the slime creates a mortar that seals most of the water on one side.

Despite your admiration for nature's work, you continue your mission to disassemble the dam. With each piece removed, more and more water comes rushing past. At the bottom, the stones are large, heavy and slick. They seem to be almost designed to be difficult to lift. With a bit of effort, you are still able to move them. Throughout the process you realize you would probably be sweating if the water was not cooling you off.

Finally, you go to lift the last stone from the stream and place it on the bank. As you first touch it, a shape explodes from beneath the stone and rushes down the river. Your initial thought must have been wrong, you suppose. Fish must swim in this river.

You move the rock, and take a moment to appreciate the strength of the current as it rushes past you. You feel a sense of accomplishment. Looking up for the first time in several minutes, you see that the clouds have broken and the sky is now clear.

But there is no sky behind the clouds.

What you thought would be the sky is actually a dome of rock. You are not standing in a valley on the other side of the mountain, but instead a massive cave within it. The most bizarre part of this development is that the cave is still lit as though there were a sun within it. Ambient light shines from all around, though you cannot identify the source. Above you, stalactites hang like icicles of rock. Unlike most of the caves you have ever seen, there is vegetation growing on this ceiling. Vines and vibrantly colored flowers hang from these stone rafters and are bathed in the strange pervasive light. Confused as you are by how it works, you are helpless but to appreciate its beauty.

Eventually you come out of your state of awe and remember that you are still standing in the stream. You need to look for a way out of this cave. You climb out, back onto its bank. You resume your walk up the stream for a few more minutes, before you come upon a log from a felled tree. All of the other trees you have seen have been alive and healthy. You want to know what could have knocked one down.

Upon closer inspection, the exterior of this log is still fairly sturdy and smooth, but its interior has been carved away. Feeling the edges of this hole in the wood, they feel rough, unlike the work of a carpenter. There is also no charring, ruling out a fire or lightning strike. As you continue with your investigation you happen to roll the log onto its side, and you realize that it would make a suitable raft. You look downstream to see that the current could carry you far out of eyesight. Excited by the prospect of no longer needing to walk, you board your natural canoe and set sail.

The water ferries you through the valley, or cave, or whatever it is. The stream bends and drops as it seems to almost be giving you a tour of its home. First you are led past a great sheer rock face. It is impressively flat and smooth, as though a slice had been cut out of the rock by some massive knife. The rock is red, like all the others in this area, but this particular face is darker in color and has a few discolorations randomly placed throughout. As you get closer, you can see that these are not natural colorings on the rock, but instead are some sort of primitive drawings carved into its maroon face.

There are some drawings of a large, terrifying looking creature. On another part of the wall are many characters of an alphabet you do not recognize. Most surprisingly, there is what appears to be a large, detailed map of the human body. At once you are excited and terrified. Have you discovered some ancient tribe of people? Was a more modern society formed in this strange place? Would they welcome you, a stranger in their lands? What on earth is that creature in their drawings, and why does it seem so menacing?

There is little time to dwell on these drawings, however, as the current quickly moves you to your next scenic view of the valley. This area is a lush, wide open plain.

With no particular sights to look at, your mind wanders. What on earth is this place? At every turn some new and ridiculous feat of nature seems to await you. It seems unlikely that the Glowing Woman is magic. It seems even more unlikely for the exit to that tunnel to have simply disappeared. Most unlikely of all is the glowing ceiling of this cave. Maybe you have discovered some new source of natural light. Maybe it will be named after you and your legacy will live on forever. Or maybe you are just deluding yourself. Regardless, your main focus is finding a way home. All of this means nothing if you are stuck here forever.

After moving for some time through this flat area, you come upon a small hill. Unlike the rest of the valley, this hill is barren and jagged, seeming out of place in an area brimming with life. The hill grows more and more narrow as it rises from the ground, and from a distance it appears to come to a perfect point at its peak. Sitting on this peak, though, is the true wonder.

At the top of this hill, sitting perfectly balanced, is a boulder the size of a truck. It appears to be the type of boulder one might see a hero lifting and throwing in a comic book to demonstrate his strength. And it is resting perfectly still on this exceedingly small point. The feat seems as unlikely as balancing a baseball on the head of a pin.

Your mind is filled with the image of yourself walking to the top of the hill and touching the rock with the smallest amount of force in your pinky finger. The rock shifts slowly at first in the opposite direction of your finger, and then in a flash it is gone, using all of its weight to barrel down the hill.

You snap yourself out of that daydream. You hope that you would never try to ruin such a beautiful display. The sight of this stone only further convinces you that there must be an advanced culture here. You cannot imagine a way in which nature would have been able to create this arrangement on its own. Then again, this valley does appear to be full of the unlikely and unthinkable.

After passing the hill, the plain resumes and fills your vision again with thick green grass. The trees continue to sway in the breeze, though less violently than during the earlier storm. There is a relaxed movement about them now, like they are slow-dancing on a green stage.

Suddenly you feel a bump, and your raft rocks back and forth in the water. A stone from below must have struck the underside of the log. You stare down into the water to check the damage, but find none. You scan the water, feeling like you are missing something. In the reflection, you can see the wooden raft, the dome of rock with all of its vegetation dangling, a few clouds drifting lazily about.

And then it dawns on you. You do not see yourself. There is no reflection of yourself in the water. You look at your hands and feet, touching them to each other, just to be certain that you are really here. Confident that you are not dead, and reminding yourself that you are not a vampire, you note this as the most bizarre part of what has already been an extremely strange journey.

Your attention is drawn away from the water only when you notice a bright light shining just beside the stream. This is noteworthy mostly because the light in this valley appears to come from no specific source, so any one point being brighter than the next seems unlikely. You raise your head to look at what you assume will be the Glowing Woman again. You mentally queue your questions like a soldier loads his gun, ready to fire at the first opportunity.

No one is standing beside the river, however. You come to find that the light that caught your eye only seems bright relative to its surroundings. The light is originating at the ceiling of the dome, and then shining down through a small opening in the roof of a shallow cave. The result is an almost angelic glow of light shining down on some vegetation within this cave. Upon closer inspection, you come to see that the only life in this dark spot lies within the ray of light. With no sun to rise or set, this small area is the only one within the cave to receive any light, and therefore is the only one capable of any growth. Surrounding this patch lies nothing, merely the rocks that make up the cave's walls.

Within the light, though, is a bouquet of colors and energy. Lush moss provides a base for a surprising variety of flowers, each with its own color and shape that you have never seen before. You are only afforded a brief glimpse, but you can see tie-die tulips, bright green roses, a small bonsai tree with purple leaves. Little dots of light dance all throughout the cave, providing a bit of light to its crevasses.

Just then, a gust of wind rolls through the valley and manages to charge its way into the cave. On its way back out, it carries with it what appear to be seeds from a dandelion, only these seeds are not the traditional white. All around you, pink seedlings float in the air, shining boldly in the light. They swirl about you, outlining the usually invisible wind, and almost appear to want to carry you along the breeze with them. Then, just as soon as they appeared, the seeds are gone. They rush away from you and up the sides of the cave around you, ready to quietly colonize whatever patch of land they happen to land on.

You are reminded of the saying, "Go wherever the wind takes you". You have never seen that mentality truly put into practice before now, and it looks like a peaceful experience. You think that if you were lighter than air, like those seedlings, you would let yourself go and join them.

You watch the path of the seeds until they are nothing but specks against the red rocks above you. By the time you realize where you are, you can hear water rushing. A glance forward shows you another tunnel. The river has not been aimlessly wandering, but instead heading towards a destination. In front of you lies pitch dark hole in the wall of the valley. It appears to be similar to the one that you entered to arrive in this valley, only this time you are given little choice on entering it or not. The current brings you quickly towards its mouth, and the banks of the stream appear steep enough on either side that climbing out would be impossible. So instead, you follow the ideals of those seedlings, and allow the current to take you where it will.

You sit back and prepare for this new unknown. You cannot see where the water is taking you, but the sound of rushing water is unmistakable. You believe that you are headed towards some kind of underground waterfall. You rock your wooden vessel back and forth in the water, proving to yourself that it can hold up under such conditions. Satisfied, you take one final glance around the valley. You appreciate its brightly colored plants, its lush greenery, and the red rocks holding them all in place. You take a deep breath and attempt once more to peer into the cave.

You can still see nothing. You are oddly unconcerned by this mystery. This cave feels less worrisome than the one that brought you into this valley, though the stakes feel much higher. On some level, you think you will survive whatever awaits you on the other side. You have to.

As you pass through the threshold of the cave, you appear to enter into a fairly complete darkness. The only sense that remains useful to you here is your hearing, and the sound of water ahead of you is growing louder. The cave smells damp and clean, but that knowledge does very little to help predict where you are headed.

The roaring of the water is still growing louder.

As the light behind you fades, you notice that the cave is not completely dark. Perhaps you are imagining it, but you seem to notice a dull pinkish glow ahead of you. It is still too dark to see where you are headed.

This is the loudest the water has been yet.

You grip the sides of your wooden raft and feel how solid it is, which calms you down. It has grown damp and slightly spongy throughout your maritime journey. You imagine that a slab of wood this size will almost certainly survive anything this cave can throw at it.

Louder still.

You are holding onto the wood for dear life. At this point the anticipation is the worst part. Maybe you were wrong about the waterfall.

The roar is deafening now.

Maybe this is just the stream increasing speed. It certainly wouldn't be the strangest thing you have seen in this valley.

Somehow even louder.

You relax your grip. It has been too long, you think. There is no way there could be a waterfall this deep into a cave. The rationalizations fly through your head at breakneck speeds.

Then you feel the drop.

Cavern

As it turns out, you are right that there is no water-fall this deep in a cave.

This is more of a rapid.

The stream dips and the water accelerates a bit, causing your vessel to accelerate as well. You briefly try to open your eyes, but close them quickly as it is still too dark to see. The water splashing around causes a mist to rise up, which you then fly through. It feels cool on your face, and soon you come to realize that you are soaked. You think that you might as well have jumped into the water and swam.

Your trip ends quickly, and the water slows down to a trickle. Your canoe comes to a lurching stop, and you take on a good amount of water as you topple back and forth in the vessel. You open your eyes, steady yourself, and immediately begin checking it for leaks or other damage. Most of the bark was scraped off, and a chunk was taken out of one of the sides, but it seems as if your raft will still float. Only, it appears to be pink. As a matter of fact, everything around you is pink. Beneath the water you can see the source of the color.

Bright, pink light originates in patches at the bottom of the river you are floating through, and the water diffuses it throughout the cave. The light ripples and flutters with the water's movements, as though the light is a puppet and the water is the master. At first you assume that this is the work of some sort of intelligent race, but then you have another thought. You run your hand through the water. As it moves, the hand remains visible to you through the crystal-clear water. Just after you disturb an area of water, that area begins to glow in the same way as the other patches below. This is some sort of bioluminescence; tiny glowing organisms that shine in turbulent water. The currents must be stirring up these small eddies of light.

The walls of the cave are all smooth stone, no doubt worn down by years and years of currents passing by them. You can faintly tell that they are grey, with veins of white running through. The glow of pink catches the white streaks particularly and makes them glow as if they are filled with neon gas. The darkness of the grey rock around them only further enhances their hypnotizing brightness by contrast.

All along you on the sides of the cave sit small, shallow pools. These tiny bodies of water are much dimmer than the river, but flash every so often with life. You debate getting out of your vessel so that you could check if there are tiny fish causing the flashes, but decide against it. If you were to lose your little raft, you would be forced to swim the rest of the way. Better not to risk it.

As you move down the stream the current begins to pick up again, and you begin to notice more and more stalagmites rising up from the floor of the river. The current bobs and weaves to avoid these rock formations. The whirlpools that form just behind the stalagmites drive the bioluminescence wild, and the result is a swirling light show that features only shades of pink. The closer you look, the more wonder you feel.

The first eddy is surprising; a tornado of light that nature seems to be creating on a whim. The next, you become amazed at the center of the vortex. It shines the brightest of any area in the water, with the area around it becoming dimmer as the water spirals outwards. It seems like a pink sun, with its rays radiating all around it. The third eddy causes you to look more closely at the water within it. If you focus for long enough, you can see small dark spots against the bright pink backdrop. This must be some pieces of rock or vegetation being washed through the river with you. You become entranced with the idea of being one of those dark specks, getting to bathe in pink light. You imagine it feels weightless, as though the light completely frees you from gravity. You are brought back from this daydream by another eddy, this one the dimmest of them all. You bring your face so close that drops of water splash up onto your face. Though you still cannot see your own reflection, you imagine these droplets glow pink on your face for a few beautiful moments before fading back to the unassuming clearness of water.

As you look closely at this new eddy you can see the individual specks of light glow within it. These are the creatures that light the cave, who seem to only exist to provide wonder to this tiny ecosystem. It must be a glorious power to be able to light the darkness like this. Chaos, though challenging, can produce a kind of beauty that we humans will never be able to capture.

For a long time, you content yourself with these small performances by the water, choosing to not think of the uncertainty you will find when this river runs its course. Your attention wanders throughout the cave.

You stare at the roof. It has smooth ridges carved through it, running in a direction perpendicular to the flow of the water. You assume that the water reached all the way up to this ceiling at one point, and these grooves were its work.

Out of the corner of your eye you think you see a shadow, or some human-like figure in the dark. Your attention snaps to the area, but it is not lighted by the pink water. This spot lies just behind a particularly large stalagmite. You stare at it for a long time, hoping to discern some movement. The shadows seem to shift and swirl. You are unable to tell if you have company in this cave, or if your eyes are simply playing tricks on you. Maybe this is an accomplice of the

Glowing Woman, silently watching and waiting to silence you for good. But you can see no features in the shadows, and soon you pass by the spot.

Giving up, you turn your attention to the floor of the cave. It looks to be made of fine sand, glowing vaguely from the light in the water. The sand shifts from the currents, giving the appearance that it is almost alive.

You are so hypnotized by this movement that you almost do not hear the splash coming from that large stalagmite. You just manage to catch a glimpse of something dark shooting up the stream ahead of you. You are immediately reminded of the dam in the valley. You look back in the shadow that you had been searching before, and find no figure there. Perhaps you are not alone.

Paranoid, you sink lower into the raft. Its sides give you some amount of comfort, and from behind them you scan the banks of this subterranean river for other shadows. The movement of the lighted water heightens your nerves even further. With each ripple in the water you flinch slightly.

In your intense focus, you realize how silent this cave is. Never before have you felt such overwhelming quiet. Even the running water that carries you makes no noise as it slides along the rocks that surround it. The only noise that fills the space are the periodic drops of water that fall from the roof. Every few seconds, a small droplet gathers enough courage to dive down and join the rest of its kind in the river below.

As it finally splashes to its destination, the noise of its arrival echoes through the cave, reverberating off of the smooth rock walls and ceiling. It seems to be a small celebration from the river water, ecstatic that their prodigal son has returned. When the echoes fade, silence returns.

You stave off your fear of the shadows for a while by counting the seconds between the drops. After enough drops, you begin to feel like the silence works in perfect symmetry with the noise. As the sound of the drip fades, the silence moves in to seamlessly fill its place. In this way they seem to bleed into one another, as though they were working together on some sort of symphony. You keep counting the seconds between the drops, fascinated to see if there is a pattern. Your study does not last long, though, as the noise of the echoes is soon drowned out by the roaring of water.

You can hear this waterfall before you ever really see it. It lies around a bend, and before long you notice a strong pink glow coming from that direction. As you round the curve in your makeshift canoe, you are shocked by the brightness of the area just ahead. It appears to be the top of some sort of wild eruption of water, and the bioluminescence goes wild in its spray. The tiny organisms jump and writhe like they have been waiting for your arrival for a hundred years, and the time has finally come. The pink color explodes out from the base of the spray, a spot so bright and vibrant that you struggle to look at it for more than a moment through squinted eyes.

You do not truly believe that this is a waterfall. Your experience since entering this cave has been mostly slow and peaceful, and that gives you confidence that the rest of your journey will remain that way. You continue to feel confident until you look just beyond the spray of pink light.

There is a flat rock wall.

Panic begins to set in again. A waterfall is now your best chance at survival. You just want to avoid some sort of underground river that will suck you under and never release you. Briefly, you debate disembarking and swimming to one of the nearby rocks. You abandon this thought quickly though, since you still most likely would have no way out. So instead, you breathe deeply. In, and out. In, and out. In, and out.

As you grow closer to the falls, you become enveloped in pink light. You feel panicked, and question your decision to stay in the tree trunk vessel. With only a few dozen feet before the fall you take in your surroundings again.

The width of the cave has narrowed, creating a funnel pointing towards the fall. The rock no longer has any semblance of a greyish color, having been completely washed out by the brightness of the pink falls. Looking up, there is a massive stalactite hanging down from the roof of the cave. There were a few others along your underground journey that you could remember, but none this size. If you were standing, it would be slightly longer than you are tall. It is also a strange structure, being very narrow at the top and very wide and bulbous at the bottom. It takes on the appearance of a speed bag that a giant boxer might pummel, though this one might shatter even a giant's hand. It has no streaks of white rock running through it like the other stone in the cave. Instead, it is one solid chunk of grey. Or at least, you assume it is grey. The pink color from the water dulls your sense of sight quite a bit.

You conclude your inspection of the rock only to realize that you are mere feet from the spray of water signaling the start of the falls or river or whatever lies ahead. It is too late to turn back. You take another deep breath. In, and out. And you prepare for what is to come. You grip the sides of your vessel hard, so you do not become separated from it. The wood has grown soft from the water, and allows you to sink your fingers into it a bit for a better grip. You close your eyes, though the brightness of the light still pushes through your eyelids. You take one last deep breath as you begin to feel the spraying water sprinkle onto your face.

In...

You gasp as suddenly you are in free fall. The light is gone, and your only tether to the outside world is the tree trunk that you clutch with white knuckles. The water splashing onto you feels more solid than liquid at speeds like this. The only sound you can hear is the air rushing past. It drowns out even the sound of the water, which you are sure is deafening in its own right.

At some point during your descent you feel your boat turn slightly to the left, and you are comforted that the water must still be guiding your raft somewhat. The descent seems to take hours, though you know that this is only because you spend every moment of it worried that it will be the last. You decide to lay down along the bottom of the vessel, to avoid any low hanging rocks that might be waiting in your path. You make a mental note that log-flume rides at theme parks are far tamer than the true experience.

When you and your raft reach what you feel to be the speed of sound, you feel the angle of descent begin to change. You are leveling out, and you gain hope that this could mean an end to the falling.

The actual end is much more abrupt and violent than you expected. In this regard, the log-flumes in theme parks around the world are fairly accurate. The raft reaches a pool of calm water, and lurches hard to stop. As a result, you roll forward within it and its nose dips down again, taking on water. You panic and lean back to stop the process, but already the raft is half full.

You are concerned about sinking for only a moment, at which point you realize you can see the water in your raft. And it isn't bathed in a pink light. Stunned, you look up to see a light beckoning at the end of the long tunnel.

Plain

The river carries you out of the cave and into the sweet sunlight. The warmth wraps around you like a towel and dries you off after your virtual bath in that waterfall. Though the sensation is nice to the skin, your eyes resist the invasion of the sun. They are still adjusting after spending so much time in the dark. You blink over and over, balancing a desire to look around with an even deeper desire to not burn out your retinas. In the meantime, you allow the sun to warm your deeply chilled body. After about ten or twenty or thirty blinks, the brightness and your eyes strike an agreement and you can take in your surroundings.

All around you lies a vast expanse, with green hills rolling out as far as the eye can see. The sky is clear blue, without a cloud in sight. These are all of the details that you notice before your makeshift raft begins to sink. It went through a beating in the caves, and it's no surprise that it could support you no longer. You hastily roll out and swim to shore, stopping only to watch the piece of wood rush away with the current. You silently thank it for carrying you this far.

You pull yourself onto the shore and restart the process of allowing the sun to dry you. All you feel is a cool breeze. The sensation would be extremely pleasant if not for the water soaking you, and instead it reduces you to shivering. Luckily, the breeze changes quite rapidly, and gives brief moments of pause before deciding on a new direction. In these moments you are allowed to be warm.

As you withstand the wind, you inspect the plains before you. The color palette of this region is all cool greens and blues. Below the horizon, a few flowers dot the landscape, adding touches of yellow and white. Certain areas produce grass of a dark, forest green hue. Other areas provide grass nearing the territory of lime green. Even staring carefully, you see no patches of brown or beige. The grass appears to be not only growing, but thriving. The whole vista looks like it could be in a lawn-care commercial. A few areas seem to hold a small quarry of greyish-purple rocks, but the rest of the area seems to be completely clear of any obstructions. Just open space all around.

Above the horizon, not a single cloud can be found. Not even a wisp that wishes it could one day grow up to become a real cloud. In the center of this sky, directly above you, the color is a dark blue. The color looks as though a magical being took the ocean, ironed out its wrinkles and rough edges, and stretched it out above you like canvas on a board. As the sky moves away from you, the color grows lighter and lighter, until near the boundary of your vision you can see that it fades from light blue to soft white. Where the sky and the plain meet to the right of you, as far out as your eyes can manage, you see something that resembles a chain of mountains. From this distance you can tell very little about them, only seeing their jagged grey outline. In its hazy lack of definition, that area seems like someone coarsely ripped off the last bits of sky that were supposed to touch the horizon.

The sun hangs at the opposite side of the valley from the mountains. You imagine that this direction is the East, and that the sun has just recently risen. It is bright and full, though maybe bigger than you remember. It bears down on you and wraps you in its warmth, and for the first time since the Glowing Woman entered your room, you feel like you are in a familiar place.

You come out of your observation to realize that many minutes must have passed, because you are completely dry and warm. With this process complete, you decide to walk away from the river and toward the chain of mountains in the distance. They appear to be the only tall structure in this plane, and you hope that from their higher elevation you might be able to see some town or civilization. You begin the long walk to your destination with hope.

The most notable characteristic about the wide-open expanse is how descriptively the grass reflects the movement of the breeze. Before any gust can reach you, it can be seen in the distance gliding across the plains, reminding you of attending baseball games as a child and watching the hitter make contact with the ball a moment before hearing the crack of the bat. The wind disturbs the grass, and causes it to ripple as though it is a great wave in an ocean of green. The movement causes the light to hit the grass differently, and therefore gives the grass the momentary appearance of having changed colors. In this way, the plains are making visible what is usually invisible to the human eye. The scene is picturesque to the point that you find yourself half expecting a nun to dance over one of the hills, singing about their beauty.

The visual aid of the grass points out an interesting detail of the gusts that glide over the plains. They last for only a few moments, always blowing in one direction, then pausing, then blowing for a few moments in the opposite direction, and pausing again. The breeze also lasts consistently longer in one direction. As the wind moves from your right side to your left, it blows for only a few dozen seconds. When the air changes direction, however, the gusts last for two or three minutes.

In this way, the wind reminds you of a restless sleeper. It tosses and turns from one side to the other, hoping to find comfort and the relief of sleep. Just as it begins to grow comfortable on its one side, the wind grows restless and decides to make a change, and the process repeats itself over and over. It favors one side slightly more, though even then it is helpless to stick to its choice when discomfort creeps up.

You walk slowly to your destination. You have no

deep desire to rush to the mountains off in the distance. You have no idea how long you will continue to journey through these strange lands, and feel like you should conserve your energy. Just as you begin to drift off into thought, you hear a familiar voice.

"You are not headed in the right direction."

You turn to find the Glowing Woman, standing tranquilly behind you. Your reaction is hardly as calm, though, as you immediately begin trying to call forward the list of questions that you have developed throughout your journey. A new one takes precedence, however.

"And why would I take directions from you? You're a weird looking woman who broke into my bedroom, kidnapped me, and left me on the side of a mountain to die!"

"Believe me, when I brought you here, I had the utmost faith that you would survive," she says. "You really must learn to trust me." She smirks as she utters the last sentence, like she has done in response to most of your questions. It infuriates you.

"Is this some sort of game to you?" You are yelling now. "Do you take some sort of sick pleasure in watching me suffer through constant panic? Trust you? To be entirely honest with you, I'm beginning to lose trust in my own eyesight! I don't even know what you are, what your name is–"

"Would it help if I had a name?"

You are caught off guard by her response. She does not smirk, nor does she respond in a mocking tone.

This is the first time that you feel as though the Glowing Woman is not trying to play with her food. You notice now that she is not glowing as strongly as the last time you saw her, or perhaps she simply seems dimmer in comparison to the bright environment around you both. It is for this reason that you can take in a few more details about her appearance. She has freckles on her face and shoulders, and her hair is sprinkled with gold.

"Well... yeah," you finally respond, "but now I feel like you're just going to make one up to keep me happy."

"You can call me Brioxa," the Glowing Woman responds calmly. Again, there appears to be no hint of sarcasm or bemusement in her voice. Perhaps you are beginning to get somewhere.

"Okay then, 'Brioxa'. If you're so knowledgeable, then what *is* the right direction?" You supplement her lack of sarcasm with your own, seeking to express how little you trust her still. Once again, the look of bemusement returns to her face.

Brioxa silently points out, just to the right of the mountain chain. Initially, you see nothing. But then, miles away you can make out a greyish dot on the horizon. It looks like an old wooden building. A barn perhaps? More important than what it looks like, is what it represents. Society! Some culture, some human hands must have built that structure, and they may be able to lead you out of this strange place.

"I can't believe it! I might survive this after all!", you

say as you turn back to face Brioxa. But she is gone. You chuckle at this, and remark to yourself that you were not entirely wrong about the Glowing Woman. She is still rude.

For the first time on your journey you become aware that the light around you is fading. The sun is moving with surprising speed across the sky above you. Your initial guess must have been correct, and the place where you first saw the sun is the East. But it inches closer and closer to the mountains in the West now.

You head out toward the building, moving at a very brisk pace. You want to reach your destination before the sun sets. Your pace only quickens as the temperature drops at the same speed as the sun. Soon your teeth begin to chatter, and goosebumps rise on your skin. You rub the sides of your arms to keep your blood flowing.

To take your mind off of the chill in the air, you try to focus on the beautiful sunset happening around you. As the mountains begin to mask the sun, their shadows extend over the plains, quickly reaching you and a few minutes later stretching on across the plain. The sky abandons its hues of blue, opting instead for an explosion of color. Streaks of pink and orange cut their way across the sky nearest to the sun. Further away from that focal point, more odd colors pop up. Various shades of deep blue, bright purple, and even bottle green hang in the air. The entire sky looks like a painter's palette after the oils have been mixed.

Luckily for you, the sight is sufficiently distracting and you forget all discomfort for a little while. By the time you reach a mile's distance from your destination, the sun drops fully below the mountains.

You are now shivering uncontrollably as you walk. The wind is cold and still ever-changing. Though, if it was a wild frenzy before, the direction of the wind seems more consistent now. The wind slowly builds to a swell in one direction, and then dissipates just as slowly. Only when the air has become perfectly still does the breeze begin again, slowly building in the opposite direction. These are the things that one notices when they are freezing in an open field, with shelter within eyesight, but still mind-numbingly far away.

It takes you only one or two eternities to traverse that last mile. Due to the all-encompassing darkness, you cannot tell much about the structure until you get within a few feet of it.

The building stands tall and cylindrical. The foundation is perfectly round and made of stone, meaning a fairly advanced people must have constructed it. The exterior is wrapped in dozens of dark wooden shingles, save for the periodic interruption of a few windows. As your gaze reaches the top you feel surprised. Four massive arms extend out from the very top of the building, all at right angles to one another. Somehow, in your shivering, you had not noticed this large pinwheel shape as you approached. The arms turn faster and slower as the wind changes direction. At times its motion is helped by the gusts, while at others the wind slows the spinning. It would appear as though you have stumbled upon a windmill in the middle of this field.

As you finally come up to the front door, you are struck by a realization. No light appears to be coming from the building. What if someone is locked away in there and not accepting visitors? Or worse yet, what if the place is abandoned altogether?

A particularly strong breeze hits and you decide that standing around debating your options will get nothing done. Trying your luck, you reach for the doorknob. And what do you know, the door is open.

Windmill

You open the door to find complete darkness. You step in but leave the door open, in case you need to make a quick exit. You allow your eyes to adjust.

"Hello?" you call out into the void. "Is anyone here?"

You wait silently, hoping to hear at least the faint sound of footsteps coming to investigate the commotion. You worry that you will be seen as an intruder, wishing to harm someone, so you would like to make yourself self as non-threatening as possible. Making sure that the owner of this windmill is aware of your presence is a good start. After a few minutes of paralyzing silence, you try again.

"I'm a lost traveler just looking for some shelter for the night. I don't mean any harm, and would really appreciate some help."

Nothing.

You strain your ears to listen for even the softest sound that might tell you if you are in the company of another. You flinch visibly with each creek of the wooden structure, shifting under the pressures from the wind outside. Finally, you grow impatient and de-

41

cide to press your luck. Hopefully this wasn't some trap set up by the Glowing Woman.

"Okay," you yell even louder than before, "I'm going to move around the house now. If you can hear me, I'm not looking to steal anything or hurt anyone. I'd just like a place to rest."

Once again receiving no response, you take your first cautious steps into the living area and close the door behind you. Your eyes have now adjusted to the darkness of the room. You can see that it is a large room with no furniture. Across from you, there is a flat wall that runs the width of the room, about 20 feet across. The wall behind you wraps around and connects with the flat wall, making the whole room the shape of a half-circle. The only noteworthy feature you can see is a staircase along the wall to your right. The staircase spirals up the curved side of the windmill. You decide that you will take your exploration upstairs, hoping to find some indicator that someone lives here.

You walk with your back to the curved wall of the room, paranoid that you might be caught off-guard by a person wishing to defend themselves from an intruder. As you make your way, you notice strange rectangles etched along the walls. Could it be some sort of pattern or artwork? You can't be sure in this darkness. As you slide your hands over each shape you feel a singular bump within its borders. All other parts of the wall feel completely smooth. You make note of this only to distract yourself from the terror of something jumping out at you from the darkness. Finally, you reach the stairs.

As one might expect, each step up the wooden planks creates an explosion of creaks and groans. Each decibel weighs on your already weary nerves as you inch your way throughout this house of potential horrors. You pause after the wood settles beneath your feet, and sharpen your focus again to detect signs of life. Invariably, you hear nothing, and begin the cycle again.

After your tenth long pause, you lift your foot to ascend further. You instead hit your head on a surface above you. What could this be? Could this staircase have led you into a ceiling? You grope with your hands, hoping to find some sort of information. Finally, your hand feels a cool, round protrusion. It seems to be able to rotate slightly on its axis, so you turn it. A small click flies through the air, and suddenly the surface above you is movable. Gently, you push upwards on it, and continue to walk up the stairs. You look around, and a wave of relief washes over you.

Light!

Beautiful pale beams of light float in through the windows and allow you to rely on more than just your senses of touch and hearing. Forgetting your desire to remain as quiet as possible, you run up the remaining stairs to the nearest opening and look out. You barely hear the thud behind you as you leave the stairwell.

At the window, you see a massive, pale blue moon

has risen just over the mountains and now bathes the plain in light. The grass ripples softly in the breeze, and the boulders reflect some of the moon's light back at you.

Believing that your luck has finally turned, you confidently turn back to the room to investigate it. You do not find much. The room is dusty and empty, and semi-circular just like the last. Near its curved wall, a staircase ascends to the next level. On the floor, you see that the previous staircase had a trap door covering its top. When closed, the door would lay flat and become of part of the floor. But now it is flung open, laying on the side of the portal that leads down to the first level.

All along the walls are the same strange rectangles that you thought you noticed in the first room. You get closer to inspect them and find that these are all discolorations in the paint on the wall. Given their size and shape, you think they must be the remnants of picture frames that have since been removed. The small indents you felt seem to be nail holes. Someone must have lived here for a long time for such drastic change to occur. All along the floor you see similar patches, but much larger. There must have been furniture in this room once, but it is all gone now.

Despite the signs that someone once called this place home, the thought of someone living here seems impossible to you now. This room is barren, and the atmosphere uninviting. Far from making the windmill seem lived in, the discolorations on the floor and walls make each room appear even more empty. The memory of each piece of furniture makes you realize just how little there is in this place now.

Just then, you hear a noise come from behind a door on the opposite side of the room from the window. The jolt of sound makes you jump. You slowly make your way across the room to confront the sound. Rationalizations begin to pop up in your head.

It must have been a broom falling off a shelf.

Maybe a small animal is trapped in there.

You reach out, praying that this door might be locked and you might be able to walk away with your blissful ignorance. Sadly, the handle rotates.

As you pull back the door, light from the moon gradually flows into what you see is a small closet. The light from the moon bathes almost the entire closet, but then skips a patch of the wall. You move to the side, assuming that your body is blocking the light. But the Shadow stays still, and then shifts suddenly to the corner. You stare for a few seconds to be sure that your eyes are not failing you, but then the Shadow flinches again.

"Hello?" you say softly, hoping to not startle this strange creature. What appears to be some sort of head turns to look up at you. A dull hum resonates through the air like an electric charge.

"I didn't mean to startle you," you console. "I'm lost and I was just looking for a place to get warm."

As you finish your sentence you reach out your

hand as a peace offering to convey your good intentions. After all, who knows if it even speaks English.

For a moment the Shadow seems to move its head to inspect your hand, but then it lashes out. You pull back your hand, shocked at how much the blow stings. The buzzing in the air intensifies. Not only do you hear it, but you feel a sensation like your whole body falling on pins and needles. Looking at your hand, you can see that the Shadow left a dark mark behind. The skin where it touched you seems dimmer now. You fear for your own safety. The Shadow's form seems to shift. It may be more agitated now.

"Wait! Wait!" you plead. "I don't want to hurt you!"

You force your voice to take on a more comforting tone. You don't want this creature to see you as a threat.

"It's okay, I'm a friend. Everything is going to be okay."

The Shadow's form softens for a moment, and you think that you may have gotten through to it. The buzzing calms slightly. But then the shape tenses up, and in a swirl of motion the Shadow flies past you and down the stairs. You hurry to follow it, but realize that you won't be able to see it in the windowless first floor of this building. You decide to check outside instead, to see if it left the house or not. You move to the window and catch a glimpse of a Shadow moving along the moonlit plain. You track it for a few moments before it disappears into a dark patch beneath a cloud.

You take a deep breath and attempt to process this new information. As it turns out you are not alone in this bizarre place. Now you know that a disgruntled shadowy creature is lurking. The thought is far from comforting.

You approach the next flight of stairs with a renewed sense of caution. The creaking now is not your concern, but all of the dark corners instead. The stairs ascend in a tight spiral, and so you cannot see very far ahead. You imagine monsters everywhere, just waiting for the moment that you lower your guard.

From the level above, a soft white light shines. You climb up from the stairs and find a large observation deck. The room is empty apart from the opening in the floor for the staircase, and moonlight streams in through the windows that encircle the room. You can see the entire expanse of the plains now, lit by the moonlight. You see no end in three directions, and only the mountains rising up in the fourth. They appear to be about five miles from this windmill.

As you survey the moonlit plain, you are struck by just how alone you are. In all directions there is nothing but space. You consider that there might be times when this thought would be comfortable and relaxing to you. But not now. Now, as you seek any sign of life or hope, this space is the most overwhelming thing in the world. Then you recall the Shadow, and remind yourself that you are not completely alone.

You still have your ghosts.

Disappointed, you look back at the moonlit observation deck. All around you there are little specks of light floating carelessly in the air. You did not notice them when you first entered the room. You assume they must be lightning bugs, but cannot get a good look at one to confirm your suspicion. The little specks swirl around you, before travelling down the stairs.

But they do not enter the same stairwell that you just used to reach this level of the windmill. You find that there are actually two openings for two different staircases in the room. Looking back, you realize that all of the rooms that you entered were only half circles. Is it possible that you have only explored half of the building?

Feeling slightly more confident with the light of the moon completely lighting your surroundings, you decide to follow the little specks of light and descend to the other half of the windmill.

The stairs are about the same as the other flights that you have climbed thus far, but with the added benefit of the glow given off by the little lightning bugs. You can still see a patch of discoloration from an old picture frame every so often.

You arrive on the second level and find no windows. The room also feels much smaller than the rooms on the other side of the windmill. You notice two doors along its curved wall, and decide that you should inspect them, but carefully. You would hate to find another creature.

You open the first door as slowly as you can manage. You find a kitchen, just as dusty and deserted as the rest of the house. You look around and see a few cupboards, a sink, a small table, and two chairs. These are the first pieces of furniture that you have seen in the whole building. You walk over to the cabinets first, wanting to check to see if there is any food there. The doors creak on their hinges. You find no food, just a small collection of cups and plates.

You close the doors and walk over to the table. You run your finger over its surface and inspect the small mountain of dust that you have picked up. You repeat this process on one of the chairs, and then look around. In the moonlight, you can see the dust hanging in the stagnant air, mixing with the one or two specks of light that followed you into this room.

You walk back out of the kitchen. You check the other room on this level, and find it is less flooded with the glow of the moon than the other rooms. Because of this, you can barely see that there are many large rectangles of discoloration on the floor. These must have been a bed and other bedroom furniture. You check the closet in this room and, rather than a living shadow, find a pile of pillows and blankets. For the first time since walking into this windmill you remember how cold you are. And, now that the panic of that Shadow's attack has subsided, you feel very tired.

You pull out the bedding materials and pile them in a corner of the room. With your paranoia still not completely gone, you close the door and lock it. You lower yourself down into your cocoon of blankets opposite the door so that you might see any intruders. You feel the warmth rise up, starting at your feet and moving slowly up your legs. You rub your hands together, hoping the friction will move this process along. The warmth finally hits your torso and penetrates deep into your core. For the first time since you appeared on the side of that mountain, you let your muscles relax.

The wooden ceiling becomes your focus and try you to take stock of the day. There is no true way to make sense of it. Between these vastly different landscapes, the Glowing Woman, the Shadow, and the fact that you have no idea how you got here, there is too much to process. All you can focus on is surviving and making it back home. All of the troubles of your normal life seem insignificant now. You crave the dull normalcy of it.

Your thoughts move to the walls of the room. There are the markings of picture frames on these ones, too. You still cannot believe that someone once slept in this room every night. You wonder, if this windmill had a mind of its own, would it miss its former tenant? Would it be glad to be rid of the intruder within its walls? This train of thought carries you into a deep, dreamless sleep.

You awake feeling as though only minutes have passed. The warm, cozy feeling still impresses you, though you must have been experiencing it constantly for several hours. Never in your life have you experienced such all-encompassing comfort.

Your pleasure lasts only until you open your eyes. Immediately upon seeing the barren wooden walls of the room, you panic. You are not in a familiar place. You are not safe. You are lost and in danger. Your breathing quickens. You are going to die out here, and no one even seems to be looking for you. You wonder if they even care.

Your stream of frenzied thoughts is interrupted when you a bright light shining beneath the door.

The Glowing Woman. Brioxa. All of your misery in this place is her fault. Maybe if you can sneak up on her, you can force her to take you home.

You slink out of your pile of blankets and begin to move towards the door.

Your heart begins to beat out of your chest.

As slowly as humanly possible, you attempt to open the door. It opens a crack, and then a few inches without making a sound. By the time you have the door a full foot open, your heart is beating so loud that the sound of it fills your ears.

And then, the rusted hinges squeak. The sound lasts for only a moment, but it causes your heart to drop. You have certainly been caught. Your captor will escape now, and you will be trapped in this land for the rest of your days. Wearily, you look through the doorway to see what remains outside. Unsurprisingly, you find nothing, but the light still shines through the room. The origin of this glow appears to be upstairs, in the room with the observation deck. Maybe you can still catch Brioxa yet.

You creep silently to the stairs, and then begin to ascend them. With each new step, you begin by touching with only your big toe. Then your other toes join it, and finally the ball of your foot. Then you slowly increase the pressure you apply on the step until it becomes enough to lift the weight of your body and rise to the next step.

After repeating this process five or six times, you finally reach the point where your head can peek into the room. Your heart begins to pound again. The anticipation crushes your nerves. After a deep breath, you pop your head up and survey the surroundings.

Again, you find no Glowing Woman, but instead something much more pleasant. The sun, as it turns out, is the source of the glow that you have been chasing. That glow leads you to take in the whole vista of the plain. The sun is rising opposite the mountain range. It illuminates the entire valley evenly, with the exception of the area hidden in the shadow of the windmill. The blades turn in the wind, slightly obstructing the view on one side. Off in the distance you can see jagged, brightly colored lines. They look almost like veins full of pastels. They must be small groves of flowers.

You continue to pan the horizon until your attention is drawn to something in the air. Miles away, you see thousands of dots floating on the wind. Just like the day before, the wind appears to be swirling and constantly changing, and these colors illustrate that. From this distance you cannot tell what their population is made up of. Birds? Or perhaps petals, like the ones in that first cave? Whatever they are, the sheer number of them is impressive. Your fears now have completely melted away. For now, you consider yourself lucky to be able to witness the beauty of this plain.

Your gaze lands on a small stream that winds its way over the rolling hills of the plain. You trace its path moving away from the mountain range. It travels many miles, growing wider and wider as it goes, until finally it connects to a much larger river off in the distance. You believe that this small stream is merely a tributary of the river that you rode into this plain. This thought comforts you, as you feel like you have had company this whole time. Just before you look away, you think you see movement. You cannot be sure of it, but you believe you saw a Shadow moving up the river, towards the mountains. The thought causes you to shiver.

With your sight-seeing complete, you decide to check the rest of the house. In the light of day, the place is much less threatening. You make your way through and check all of the rooms again, hoping that you might find something that could help you get home. You find nothing but dust mites. You then remember that in your panic, you didn't check the cupboards very thoroughly last night. For the first time since arriving, you realize that you haven't eaten in well over 24 hours, yet you feel no hunger. A day might not even be 24 hours in this place, but that is a rabbit hole that you would rather not go down at the moment.

The first two or three cupboards that you check are just as empty as the rest of the house. In the cabinet below the sink, you finally find something. The first thing to catch your eye is a shiny metal tea kettle. You pick it up and dust it off. There isn't a trace of rust on it anywhere. The other object in the cabinet is a small cardboard box. The exterior of it reads *English Earl Grey*.

Tea! Finally, something that you might be able to consume. You stick the tea kettle under the faucet and turn the knob, but nothing comes out. You have tea and a kettle, but no water. After hours of consuming nothing, you feel very intent on drinking this now. So, you walk out of the kitchen, kettle in hand, to pull some water from the river.

You walk down the set of stairs nearby and find another entrance to the windmill. That doorway leads you out to the backside of the building, facing the chain of mountains. The sun warms your skin slowly, but the crisp morning air prevents the heat from becoming overbearing. You notice as you walk that your feet become wet as you step through the dew-covered grass. This sensation only furthers your thirst.

In total, the walk takes you no more than a few minutes. The babbling of the river begins as a whisper in your ear and builds as you approach. By the time you arrive, its gurgling is distinct. As a habit, you stick your hand into the water first to feel the temperature.

It is freezing cold. You set the kettle down and bring your face down to the water. You cup your hands and splash some onto your face. Immediately you feel more alert and awake than you had at any point since you arrived in this place. You grab the kettle and dip it into the water until it is full. It bubbles and glugs as the air inside is forcibly replaced with water. You stand up and turn to return to the windmill.

When you reach the kitchen, you set the tea kettle down on the stove top and set about trying to find some matches. It seems like a long shot, but in one of the top-most cabinets you find a package of them. You take one and save the rest for later. You turn the gas on, strike the match, and let the fire of the stove work its magic. While the water boils you return to the other cabinets where you found the cups last night. By the time you track them down, the whole kitchen is filled with a high-pitched whistling. You remove the kettle from the burner, place a teabag in the cup, pour some of the water into it, and sit down to enjoy.

You stare out of the window next to the kitchen table. As you drink the tea, the plan for the rest of your day unfolds. While the windmill seems like a cozy and safe place, you fear that you might be isolated from finding any sort of help from the outside world. To survive, you must go out and find help, not wait for it to come to you. That is the only way you might make it back home.

You finish your cup, and decide to walk out to the river and wash it. Then you make your way into the bedroom and fold all of the blankets, before replacing them in the closet. It seems crazy, but this place has been your shelter. You may not have survived without it. And though it seems impossible right now, perhaps someday another person will live within these chambers and call this place home. For that person's sake, you don't want to leave a mess.

With the windmill clean, you set out to find your way.

Ridge

You walk to the same small tributary that you visited earlier in the morning. On your left, there is the wide open plain that you crossed to get to the windmill. On your right, there is the ridge of mountains that has been looming over you for the past day. Not wanting to regress, you set out to the right, walking along the stream as you go. You are excited for the change of scenery, though you still worry that the Shadow could be lurking somewhere out there.

After walking for about a mile, you begin to wish that you still had that piece of driftwood that you used as a makeshift canoe. You would be moving much faster if you could be carried along by the current. With each step you take, you long for that piece of bark slightly more. Finally, you give up on this thought and look straight up at the sky.

Your mind is almost completely blank as you take in the view. There are a few clouds, moving lazily towards the mountains. You squint at one and it looks oblong, almost like a football. You try with another cloud, and this one is in the shape of a lightbulb.

Just then, something strikes your foot and the

whole world seems to flip upside down. You land on the ground with a thud, having apparently tripped over something. You look back to find another piece of wood, this one slightly larger than the last. It looks to be about three feet across and four feet long. You cannot believe your luck. Immediately you forget the soreness in the toe that you just stubbed and begin to haul the thing into the stream. It is heavy, and the process is hindered by the strong current in the water. The current catches you off-guard, since this tributary is so narrow, and you nearly fall several times as you try to wade into it.

Finally, you manage to get the driftwood into the water. You climb on and set sail. The water is indeed moving faster than it was yesterday, and you notice the mountains quickly getting larger. You decide to lean your head back and close your eyes. Though you slept soundly last night, you know that it could be a long time before you find another moment to relax.

Thoughts buzz through your head left and right. The Shadow, Brioxa, and the many sounds of the plain all jostle for your attention. You have been through a great deal since you arrived in this strange place, and it will take some doing to make sense of everything. To help this process along, you decide to name each thought as it comes up, and focus on it for a moment. Then you can allow yourself to move on, having let your mind run its course. You decide to focus on the sounds of the plain first. These are the simplest thoughts that come to your mind.

Listening.

The rushing of the water that carries you is the most prevalent sound. It gurgles and splashes beneath you, with droplets landing on your face every so often. You can hear the water slap against the few rocks lying in its path. For a while that rushing is all you can notice. Soon, though, you begin to hear of the wind again. It moves gently through the grass on the banks of the river.

Feeling.

The wind flows over your skin just like the water flows over the bed of the stream. It has resumed the pace that it moved at yesterday, with its force swelling and then quickly fading, before changing direction and repeating the process. You find the repetition soothing and familiar. All you do is feel the air for some time.

Worrying.

You cannot keep your worries silent forever. Before you know it, your mind is filled with concerns about getting home. You wonder if you will ever see your loved ones again. You wonder if you will ever smell the normal scents of your home again.

Despair.

You are all alone in a foreign land, without a soul to help you. If you consider the situation objectively, things are hopeless. Why do you even bother with this journey to nothing?

Panic.

Your muscles begin to tense, as you feel danger

closing in around you. You are sure that the horrible Shadow creature is lurking in the water, just beside you, waiting to strike. Your eyes pop open, and your fist cocks back.

"I see you!", you shout prematurely, eager to prove that you will not be beaten so easily.

But you see no creature, nor any other kind of danger, just the quiet plain. You sit back in your raft, shocked at how quickly you fell into a panic when you allowed your mind to wander.

Listening.

You sit there staring blankly at the wood making up your raft, but not taking in any of the information it provides. Instead, you return your thoughts to the breeze, and the rushing of the water.

Calming.

You cannot allow your fears to control you like that, you decide. Dwelling on such negative thoughts will bring no peace, it will only distract you from the larger goal. You must stay positive, and you must escape this place. Still, it felt good to label what your worries are. At least now you know what you are up against.

Looking further into the distance, you find yourself within a mile of the ridge. There is a lush forest starting at the base of these mountains, rising up to the top of the ridge about a mile up. The trees are so dense that you cannot see any further than a few feet into the forest. You think that you might be able to spot a village off in the distance if you can climb to the top of the ridge, though you may have a tough time getting to it. The sides of the ridge are a steep incline, and the vegetation won't help.

But then you see a break in the trees. The clearing is so neat that it seems to be a man-made trail. There is a perfect path, extending into the forest and disappearing around a bend. This may be the only way for you to quickly ascend the mountainside. While the idea of sitting safely in your new raft sounds less taxing, you decide to try your luck with this new path.

You dismount and swim to the bank of the stream. It is far more difficult than you had assumed, due to the strong current. Still you make it to the shore, with some effort, and pull yourself out of the water. Luckily, the air is warm and you dry quickly in the sunlight. By the time you complete the walk to the trailhead, it is as though you have never been in the water. You look down the path and still learn very little about it, except that it is clear. You take a deep breath, and begin to walk ahead.

There are very few sounds that penetrate the wooded area to your right and left. Within a few steps, the stream sounds as though it is miles away. A few more steps, and you cannot hear it at all.

A canopy of branches forms above your head as you continue. The path is only lit by the thin strips of light that can manage their way between the leaves. In the nearly stagnant air, the sunlight becomes a maze of crisscrossing beams. For a moment it looks like a scene in a spy movie, where you must sneak by a system of laser beams. This idea fades as you cross through the first few beams of light without any sort of alarm going off.

You stop for a moment and inspect one of the trees. It is clearly a pine, but an unusual one. Its bark is layered and scaly like the skin of a snake. As you run your finger over its surface you cut your finger on one of the sharper scales, though the wound does not bleed. The branches, at least the ones this low down, extend out for at least 8 feet. They split into smaller branches, and then smaller still as they move away from the trunk. Finally, each branch is punctuated with a mess of long, deep green needles. Each needle is exactly the same length and color, which gives them an almost manufactured look. But as you run your hand through them, you can feel that they are quite naturally made. You return to the trail, and now notice that you have not been walking upon dirt, but instead on a thick mat of needles that have fallen from their respective branches. They give the forest floor a near uniform brown texture, and crunch softly beneath each step.

The trail turns upward, and you begin gaining elevation. Though you are by no means out of shape, the steepness of the climb seems like it should be well outside of your abilities. And yet, as you continue, you do not feel winded. In fact, you do not lose your breath at any point during the ascent.

After maybe an hour's climb through the dense forest, the trees finally break. The trail opens up to a face of magnificent rock. The closest thing that you can compare it to is granite, but that does not quite represent it well to the imagination. The most prevalent color is a cool grey, but within can be found nearly every color in the rainbow, shining radiantly in the sunlight. You decide to take a break here to admire your progress and plan your next steps, as these rocks are even more steep than the trail before. You turn around to see that you have made it up almost three-quarters of a mile. In front of you seems to be about a half-mile of rock, going up at a worrisome angle. You look to your right and left in an attempt to find a more gradual path, but see rock of about the same slope. Your resolve to reach the summit of the ridge begins to shake as you peer to the top. Is there even anything at the top? You strain your eyes and notice only one, subtle movement: a shadow, ducking behind the rocks.

This could be the Shadow from the previous evening, yes, but it could also be a sign of another being. Perhaps it could even be another human! Despite minimal odds of the encounter being pleasant, the hope in this idea is all you need.

The slope is much too steep for you to walk up, as you could easily tumble backwards and injure yourself. The rocks are not so steep, though, that you must free-climb them. Instead, you decide to ascend on all fours like a bear might, not stopping lest you lose the small amount of momentum that you could build up.

You take a deep breath and get a running start before leaning forward slightly so that your hands can help steady you. The time seems to pass shockingly quickly as you wait for fatigue to hit you. Flashes of color rush past your eyes, further disorienting your sense of your surroundings. Without any semblance of cramping or soreness, you find the slope of the rock becoming more gradual. You look up and see that you are no more than 200 feet away from your destination. You are able to casually walk the last bit of the climb again, and finally you are standing on the strip of almost perfectly level ground. You are on a ridge that runs along the top of this mountain chain.

You excitedly look to see what is on the other side of the ridge, but the sight lying before you causes an immense amount of confusion. You see before you the exact plain that you had just hiked out of. Everything is familiar, down to the small purplish rocks dotting the grass. You decide that the blood must have rushed to your head as you climbed, and you must have turned yourself around. So you whirl around to see what is behind you and find, again, the same plain. You stare for a long time at the expanses, each plain lying at either side of the ridge. Everything about the two plains is exactly the same: the colors, the network of streams, and even the clouds in the sky. The only difference you can see between the two is that the valley that you just climbed out of has the windmill, while the new valley has none.

After the shock of this new discovery has subsided, you finally take the time to look along the ridge. To your right you find a line of narrow, jagged rock out-croppings that, when arranged in a row as they are, form a sort of uneven pathway that one could walk across. To your left however, you find something much more exciting.

Into the remainder of the ridge, for as far as you can see, there is a sort of staircase. It looks almost like the path atop the Great Wall of China, but carved into the ridge instead of sitting on it. You approach care-fully to inspect whether your eyes are deceiving you, but find instead only fine craftsmanship. The steps are all level and smooth. Some take the traveler fur-ther up in elevation, while some take the traveler back down, but the overall trend of the path is upwards. It must have taken some poor mason ages to make these. And then you realize: this is yet another indi-cation that there is some civilization! And these steps must lead you there.

You strain your eyes once more to try to see if you can get a glimpse of a hut or a tent or any sign that human life lies ahead. The steps wind their way up and down and up again before finally disappearing into a nebulous fog. There, at the very edge between what can be seen and what is hidden, you see a shad-owy figure slither past. The sight causes you to jump back suddenly. Surely you cannot be following the ex-act same path as this creature.

As if on cue, a familiar voice appears behind you.

"You don't need to fear it, you know."

You turn to see the glowing figure of Brioxa, smiling playfully at you. Her bemused look does little put you at ease.

"Oh really? Well it didn't seem friendly the last time I saw it," you respond.

"You merely startled it. I had hoped you would have a calming effect, but it appears that neither of you are quite ready for that."

"So you knew that a creature like that," you gesture down the path, "would be hiding in that windmill when you sent me there? Were you trying to feed me to it?"

The smirk on Brioxa's face turns into a full-blown smile at this accusation. "Feed you to it? How ridiculous a thought!" She chuckles softly to herself. "I meant for you to help it! And for it to help you."

"Well that was pretty tough to do with it screeching and running off like that. So, what is it? Can it help me get out of here?"

"In a sense," Brioxa responds, a thoughtful look covering her face.

You are beginning to grow tired of the riddles and secrets. Just as you are about to begin a long rant about her cruelty towards you, she begins to speak sternly.

"It would be in your best interest to find out that creature's nature yourself. As far as how to go about such a task," Brioxa pauses to gaze off in the direction of the steps, "I believe you can guess what you must do."

You turn to look at the ceiling of clouds you would

be walking into. While you are tired of being strung along like this, this staircase does seem to be your best hope of finding help. After a lengthy pause, you turn around to face your captor.

"Fine, but how many more trails do I have to follow before-"

Brioxa has once again disappeared without a trace. If you ever do make it out of this alive, you should leave her out of the story, you think. They would probably throw you in an asylum before they believed you.

You start on your journey up the ridge. The scale of it would have been very intimidating, were it not for your newfound athleticism. You begin climbing the stairs quickly; first one at a time, then two, then three.

After a few dozen steps you notice an odd quality of the stone. It has a rubber-like quality that softens the impact of each step, and rebounds slightly. As the staircase crests and begins to head downward for a spell, you find yourself distracted and neglect to slow down and accommodate the change. As a result, you leap downwards and skip six or seven steps in the process.

But you do not injure yourself. Instead you are launched up by the trampoline-like rock a few feet in the air. You land softly on the rock again, maybe twenty feet from where you began your tumble. You take a moment to catch your breath and evaluate your situation, and then grow excited by this new mode of transportation.

You fall often as you learn how to navigate the ridge, but soon you are bounding along it, skipping dozens of steps at a time. With each leap you worry that you will find the usual type of rock when you land. The type that would break your legs. But every landing is soft and spongy, and sends you shooting back up towards the sky. You only grow more and more bold as tall walls rise up to your right and left, making the stone staircase feel more like a narrow passageway in a castle than anything else.

Before you realize, you are in the thick haze of fog that you saw when you first reached the summit. The sky above and the plains below disappear behind a curtain of grey mist. You slow your pace a bit here, hesitant to find some unexpected cliff that you would no doubt be launched off by this odd rock. And, you must not forget, you do think you saw that terrible Shadow heading along this same path.

Because of your slower speed, you are able to notice a narrow offshoot in the rock, cut into the wall to your left. You fall and tumble along the stairs in the process, but you are able to stop and inspect it. In the stillness of the mysterious foggy ridge, you hear something bubbling.

Spring

The path is rough and provides no steps, unlike the staircase that you have been travelling along. You can see that it slopes down slightly, and then left around a bend. You cannot see what is at the end of the path, but you can hear it. The sound is relatively familiar and inviting, like the babbling of a brook or the soft bubbling of a warm tea kettle. You cannot resist taking a look at the origin of that noise.

As you descend down this new path, you inspect the rock that makes up this ridge. It is dark colored, and at first glance appears to be solid black. But after a closer look, you find that it is actually two-toned. The entire rock appears to be covered in thin stripes, half black and half dark grey. Each strip of color is no more than a quarter of an inch across.

You venture to touch the stone with your hand for the first time, and find it to be stiff, as though you are touching the hard rocks that you are accustomed to. Then, as you touch another region of the stone a few feet away, you find it just as rubbery as you had felt on your trip down the ridge. You repeat this process of poking and inspecting for some time before you finally figure out the pattern. The strips of black rock are hard, like granite, but the grey strips have properties more like those of rubber. Thus, you were able to bounce along like you had earlier, but you can still walk on the stone without feeling any tremendous difference between it and rocks you are used to.

By the time you figure all of this out, you have arrived at the end of the path. Here it opens up into a circular plateau on the side of the ridge. Looking out, you can still only see a few dozen feet in front of you before all vision is blocked by the fog.

The plateau is small, only about ten feet across of smooth rock. As you look around you see the source of the noises. A small pool of bubbling green liquid sits on one side of the plateau. You walk up to its edge and bend down to inspect it. Heat rises from the liquid and condenses in the cooler air, creating an even more dense fog just above its surface. The liquid itself is fairly clear, with only a slight green tint to it. You breathe deeply to take in its smell and find yourself inhaling something like the chlorine that one would find in a pool. Finally, you dip your hand in to check the temperature, and find it soothingly warm.

Under most circumstances, you would not enter such a strange pool filled with unknown liquids in a bizarre place. But the temperature has apparently dropped as you climbed. You did not notice it at first. You certainly worked up a sweat on your run up the ridge, and since you have cooled down from that, you now find yourself shivering. With the warmth of the pool as your only option, you carefully step in.

The interior of the pool makes the task of entering very easy. Some sort of erosion has worn away several steps along its edge that you can use to climb in. The transition is easy, and you rush to get out of the cold air. You descend until you are up to your neck in warmth, and take a deep breath. You find the process of breathing slightly difficult, though not from the air itself. The fluid of the pool is somewhat dense and forces your chest to work if it wants to draw in air.

You make your way around the pool, feeling as you go. There are many bubbles in the water, and they obscure any vision of what lies at the bottom. As you run your hand along the smooth rock lining of the pool, you feel jets of hot water coming from small holes in the stone. These must be the source of both the bubbles and the heat. The overall effect reminds you of an expensive hot tub that someone has designed very carefully to look like a natural feature.

Finally, you come to what you have been searching for: a ledge just high enough to allow you to sit without too much of your body being exposed to the elements. You raise yourself up and manage to arrange your body such that only your neck and head are out of the liquid, and the rest of you is warm below. As you lean back, you find that there is a more or less upright piece of stone that allows you to recline as though you are on a sofa.

The small jets of water now apply their heat more

directly to your skin. At first the sensation is uncomfortable, like when one first steps into a hot shower. But then a different effect begins to take hold, and your muscles relax as they would if you were receiving a massage.

The hot water is affecting multiple different areas. First, a stream of water relaxes your shoulders, which feel like they have been tense for the entirety of your time in this bizarre place. The two jets hitting your lower back work out a knot that had been residing there for a few days prior to your journey. The same can be said for the few jets affecting your legs, which had become weary from all of your travelling.

You look around the plateau and find nothing that you would consider threatening. There is some concern that the Shadow might sneak up on you here, but you feel confident that you would see it coming. At this point you decide to give yourself fully to the idea of relaxing, if only for a moment, in this unknown environment. You close your eyes, and take one long, deep breath. After you exhale, you take one more, to fully convince your body that it is time to let its guard down.

With your muscles gradually unwinding, you set your mind to taking in all of the feelings that your body experiences. The most overwhelming is the tingling of the bubbles as they swirl around you. The sensation is not so much that you feel tickled or uncomfortable in any way, just that you are aware of how lively the fluid is.

Next you allow your legs to float in the surprisingly buoyant fluid. They hover just above the shelf on which you sit. Your toes uncurl, and you wiggle them, feeling the bubbles floating through the gaps between them. You engage the muscles in your ankles, drawing small circles with your feet, and then allowing them to rest in whatever position feels most comfortable at the moment.

You notice your shin and thigh are at an obtuse angle to one another, and you can feel your hamstrings loosen as they are no longer under any pressure. The water from one jet hits your left calf, and another two apply themselves to the back of each thigh. In all cases, the muscles loosen, and soon your legs become so relaxed that the only sensation you have below your hips is that of the bubbles, hurriedly running all over your skin.

The next feeling to catch your attention is the shelf on which you sit. It is smooth, but not perfectly even, with an edge that has been rounded off by the constantly moving fluid around it. It must have taken millions of years to form.

You are slouching, so that your lower back does not touch your rocky seat. This area of your body only feels the bubbles flowing over it as well. Your abdomen rises slightly with each breath. You find it easier to draw in air this way, allowing your stomach to expand rather than your chest. Your chest itself remains still, and only moves slightly as your lungs fill with air. Your upper back rests of the side of the pool.

Again, the rock is not perfectly flat. You feel that your right side is forced slightly more forward than your left.

You divert your attention for a moment to ensure that, with each exhale, your shoulders untense a bit more. When you are satisfied that they are relaxed, you note your arms. They are raised up out of the pool, resting on its edge instead. The chill in the air that flows around them feels refreshing in comparison to the intense warmth of the water that surrounds the rest of your body.

You run your fingers over the stone around you, and take notice of the miniscule peaks and valleys on its surface. You imagine it would seem like a difficult terrain to cross if you were the size of an ant. You crane your neck around in a circle, stretching all of its complex muscles. You can feel a breeze glancing off your forehead and running through your hair.

You open your eyes and admire the landscape around this pool. There are deposits of snow all around the plateau. Much like knowing hunger only increases one's appreciation for food, the very thought of the cold enhances the coziness of this natural hot tub.

Off in the distance, you can see the outline of another part of the ridge hidden behind a wall of mist. You became fairly turned around when you left the staircase that you had been climbing, so you do not know if what you see is a place that you have been to or a place that you are going towards. In either case, you are reminded that you must continue travelling soon. You cannot simply hide here and wait to be rescued. You need to seek out help yourself.

And so you take a few more minutes to enjoy yourself before returning to the trail. The sensation that you lock in on is the bubbles swirling around your body. They give you the sense that you are floating, and weightless. What strikes you as truly extraordinary about the sensation, though, is how random it all is. Though you try, you cannot find a pattern in the swirling of the bubbles. The jets beneath you vary constantly in their intensity and heat, and the bubbles they produce move wildly through the liquid of the pool, as if desperate to ascend to the surface and be released into the air.

Under normal circumstances, such chaos would unnerve you and make you desire for order. But not here.

In this environment the entropy seems beautiful. And in this moment, every time that you have ever worried about losing control seems so foolish. Entropy surrounds the world, and to try to fight it is a waste of time. The only way to truly be happy is to appreciate the beautiful thing that is.

A speck of light catches your eye, seeming like a blur as it rushes past you. For a moment it seems like you were just seeing things, but as you look around you see that you are surrounded by light. The pool glows in this new ambiance, and the entire mountain landscape disappears behind the powerful brightness. And, just as quick as it came, the light is gone.

You sit up, craning your neck around to see if you can identify what just happened. Off in the distance, hidden slightly by a veil of fog, you can see the bright glow swirling around like a flock of birds. They are the same glowing bugs that you found in the windmill!

You watch them swirl around. There must be thousands of them floating above you. But quickly they disappear, flying away on a change in the wind. You feel sorry to see them go, but at least you were present to appreciate the beauty of their brief visit.

Feeling as though your time in the pool is up, you lift yourself out and back into the plateau around it. The mountain wind cuts through you, and you begin to shiver wildly. You think that perhaps entering the pool was not the wisest decision. You decide that you must get back to the staircase and start to run. It will both dry you off more quickly and keep your heart rate up so that you do not freeze to death.

Just before you enter the path back to the trail, you notice a golden light behind you. You spin around to see the little lightning bugs again. But you do not see anything, and in your disappointment you nearly miss it.

You look back at an outcropping towards the side of the plateau, which caught your eye. You approach, and find hanging from it a long brown cloak, with golden accents. Examining the cloth, you see that it is intricately woven, with designs and symbols stitched into it that you have never seen before. You wrap yourself in it and feel that it is thick enough to block the wind.

And so you embark along the path back to the ridge wrapped in your new cloak. You are happy, though a bit confused about Brioxa's motives in leading you along this journey.

Is she simply toying with you, or does she actually want to see you survive?

Fork

You pick up your journey along the ridge just how you left it. You take a few cautious steps, to be sure that the rock still has the same spongy quality, then push your pace. The next thing you know you are bounding along at breakneck speeds, leaping thirty feet at a time.

You cannot precisely say how much longer you continue along the path. With the fog everywhere, your sense of time falls by the wayside.

The first change you notice is the direction of the steps. During your whole hike, the ridge has been constantly rising and falling with the steps following along. But the general direction of the path had been up, towards what you hoped was a mountainside village. Now, the ridge is gradually taking you back down.

Before long, you begin to come out of the fog that had engulfed you at the outset of the hike. Between leaps, as you hang in the air for a moment before the shackles of gravity drag you back down, you take the chance to look around at the area around the ridge. To your dismay, there are no cozy huts or proud castles.

Most of what you see is foliage. The trees that you walked through at the base of this mountain range are following you along as you go. The only features of note are two bright blue lakes, one on each side of the ridge. You are reminded that bizarre mirrored landscapes border you.

The path along the top of the ridge carries you ever closer to the level of the forest floor. At the speed you are moving, the descent feels sudden and unwelcome. At least up here you feel a sense of progress. You are covering ground much faster than you would be down below, and you hope this ridge lasts forever.

Sadly, this cannot be. The path finally dips below the tops of all of the trees, and in front of you there is a dirt path. You gradually try to slow your speed, but take a false step, slipping on the springy rock. Your body tumbles forward, head over heels, until you come to a stop a few hundred feet from the end of the mountain path. Defeated, you walk the last stretch toward the firm, boring ground.

The dirt trail is still not without its interesting details. Again, you find the hints of other humans having come this way. There is little grass along your route, showing that it has been well-used. And no trees block your way, as if someone had cleared them to allow travelers to move freely. Your confidence in finding some kind of civilization builds.

The scenery itself is not so upsetting to look at. Towering pine trees border the path on both sides. In the underbrush, you can see multicolored flowers and moss growing here and there. As you continue to walk, the underbrush grows thicker and thicker.

Just as you are beginning to grow used to you new surroundings, you come to a fork in the road. This worries you. Perhaps only one will lead to civilization, while the other will lead you deeper into the wilderness. You investigate both legs of the split to see if one is more traversed, but find nothing. Just like all of the other landscapes you have seen, the right and left sides of this fork are perfect mirrors of each other.

You are very worried now, as your life could be at stake here. What if you are a mere mile from help, but choose the wrong path? You could be lost out here for another week. You could die, and then Brioxa would have what she wants.

Instinctually you look around for her, trying to find the glow of her gown. You realize that this is ridiculous. You are still not sure of her motives, so how can you look to her for direction?

With no other means of deciding, you eye both sides carefully. Both stretch out for about a mile before curling over a small hill. Both are bordered by thick lines of trees and bushes. You cannot even use the old 'path less travelled' strategy, as it appears that both are equally worn in. It would appear that you have an equal chance of finding shelter with either side.

You wish you had a coin to flip. That way if you chose wrong, you could blame an inanimate object rather than yourself.

You close your eyes and breathe deeply. The air is clean and sweet-smelling. The soft aroma of pine wafts around you, ceaselessly reminding you of the presence of the trees. The sun shines down and warms your shoulders and face. You notice that your muscles have tensed up in the stress of the decision, and you allow them to relax. You have no idea which way you are going to choose. With all that you have gone through in the past few days, you find that your mind is cluttered and messy. It is extremely difficult to decide with so much noise within your mind, so you decide to try to empty it.

You imagine your mind as a flowing river. Any time a thought pops into your head, you consider it for a moment, and then let the current take it away. You picture the river that you rode on when you first arrived in the plain. The memory of its crisp water comes back to you quickly. Then, you think of Brioxa. You imagine her pupil-less purple eyes, her long black hair, and her golden skin. You find yourself wishing that she would appear and tell you which road to take. But then you give the thought up to the current that is your mind. You continue this process with every thought you have. The Shadow, the slight ache of your feet, even thoughts of your family all flow quietly away.

Soon your mind is clear and empty. You focus only on breathing deeply. In, then holding the air in your lungs, and then out. A wave of euphoria washes over you as you experience the joy that is thoughtlessness.

As you exhale one particular breath, the wind swells. The force of the gust catches you off-guard and knocks you clean from your feet and onto the ground. You begin to pick yourself up, more convinced than ever that the environment hates you, when you notice where you have been blown to. You find yourself laying a few feet down the rightmost leg of the trail. You suppose you can take this as the clearest sign you will get, and begin to walk.

While you move down the path you look back over your shoulder, trying to take one last look at the other leg. The fork in the trail shines brightly, but you cannot tell why at first. Then you notice many yellow and white flowers surrounding you. They seem to catch the sunlight and reflect it back ten-fold. You look at one closely, and find that it is almost metallic, yet soft to the touch. A few pink and blue butterflies hover near these flowers. The vibrant colors make this area of the trail seem particularly alive.

The flowers and butterflies become less frequent as you walk, and soon they disappear altogether. Now the woods around you seem darker than before, and indeed they are. Without the flowers to catch the sun's light, the walk seems a bit dimmer. You look up at the sky and find that you can see less of it than you could previously. Maybe this is just due to the trees around you getting taller. But soon you are walking in almost complete darkness. The very tops of the pine trees seem to curl over in an effort to reach the other side of the path. The result is a canopy that the sun cannot penetrate. You briefly debate turning back, but ahead you can see some amount of light, so the canopy must come to a quick end.

But you are wrong about this assumption. The canopy remains as solid as ever, and as you approach you see that the light is a fairly unnatural glow unlike sunlight. Your heart leaps in your chest for a moment. Perhaps this is Brioxa?

You pull yourself back. Why are you looking forward to your next meeting this much? You still cannot rule out the idea that she has brought you here to kill you, and that she has just been toying with you this whole time.

Your mind is pulled off this train of thought by the source of the glow. It is not Brioxa, but a cloud of those lightning bugs. There are more of them here than you have seen at any other point during your journey. They fill the entire path with soft, ambient light. Immediately your surroundings seem warmer and inviting, like a home decorated for Christmas shining in the dark. Amidst the bugs you begin to see spots of much brighter color. The flowers are glowing now, pinks and blues and whites and yellows all popping out. Soon even the needles on the pine trees seem to be glowing a dim green.

You are astounded by the uniform glow that now surrounds you. You try to peer deeper into the forest, to see if all the plant life is behaving this way. But you cannot see much farther than a few feet into the brush. The rest of the forest is dark, and that darkness is impenetrable compared to the bright light of the path.

You choose to focus on the path instead of the darkness that lies just beyond it. Your entire field of vision is beautiful and energizing. It feels as though you may even be glowing, and you look down to check. It is hard to tell with all of the light shining around you.

You now notice the lightning bugs are swirling around you. Briefly, you consider that they may try to carry you off, as if your life had suddenly become fairy tale. But the tiny balls of light do not. Instead, they swirl around you for a few moments, and then all rush off in one direction. Your eye follows their path instinctively and find that the bugs are all swirling around a new spot now. At first you cannot tell what attracts them to this new location. Perhaps they simply swirl in random spots, and you were just lucky enough to be in the middle of one of them. But then something strange catches your attention. Some of the lightning bugs are disappearing and reappearing as they circle their new spot.

In fact, all light is blocked in that area.

Your mind becomes clear. There, silhouetted against the warm glow of the plants and at the center of the swarm of lightning bugs, stands the Shadow.

As the bugs swirl around it, you can just barely make out what the Shadow is doing. Its back is hunched over, its arms covering its head. Then it seems to flail, trying to swat at the bugs. You take pity on the thing. It seems like a scared animal trapped in a corner. You move toward the Shadow, hopeful that if you help it, you may gain its trust.

"Hey there," you try to say in the softest voice you can muster.

When you speak up the bugs disperse. This worries you, as the bugs were your main way of keeping track of where the creature stands. It takes all your focus to follow its movements, but the Shadow begins to lower its arms. It appears to look around, not completely sure of what has happened, but beginning to let its guard down.

Then it sees you.

Immediately the creature lowers itself into a crouch, which you assume is its fighting stance. You again hear a buzz resonating through the air. This must be the creature's defense mechanism. Despite this show of tenacity, it still seems scared. The Shadow flinches whenever a bug comes near it, swatting wildly at the insect before returning to its fighting stance.

One of the tiny specks of light lands on your hand, and you inspect it. These little creatures have been following you throughout your journey, but you have not been able to get such a close look at one until now. You are surprised to see that these are no ordinary insects. In fact, they seem to deny all of the laws of physics that you can think of. You can feel it as it sits on your arm, just as you might feel any bug, but the light has no definite source, and no true body. You are bewildered by this new discovery. They are, as far as you can tell, simply tiny bodies of living brightness. They are light come to life.

Then it dawns on you.

The light must harm the Shadow! When you last encountered it in the windmill, you must have exposed it to the moonlight, causing it to panic and screech. And now, too, it is being attacked by brightness on all sides. The poor Shadow must be in the midst of a never-ending wave of agony.

"I can help you!", you say a bit too eagerly.

The Shadow jumps back a step, and the buzzing sound intensifies.

"Let me lead you", you try more softly. "I can guide you into the darkness. The light won't hurt you there."

The Shadow's head appears to rise a bit. Could it be able to understand what you are saying? It stops swatting at the bugs and regards you as its hands lower to its sides. You are now no more than a few feet from the creature, and you decide to try your luck.

You step forward slowly, with your hands outstretched before you, palms upturned, in a show of goodwill. The Shadow does not step back, but instead looks you up and down. You venture to take another step, and again it stays still.

On your third step, one of the tiny specks of light crosses between you. The Shadow's concentration is broken. It regards you with apprehension, arms rising to defend itself. Its head tilts down, checking the now minimal distance between you. The Shadow looks back up at you. You feel the buzzing in the air on your skin now, and you look around to see all of the leaves vibrating slightly. The Shadow turns and runs.

"Wait!", you call out, and begin running after it.

The creature is a blur as it moves down the trail, obscuring any light that it passes by. It is difficult to keep track of it, as it remains only a silhouette rather than a physical object. Things become particularly dire as the light from the surrounding canopy fades. Soon, you are running through the darkness, attempting to catch a Shadow.

You debate giving up your pursuit. It will be impossible to find the creature in this blackness. At this point, you become convinced that it has certainly stopped and allowed you to run past, unable to see your mistake.

Just as you begin to slow down, a new light comes into view. This one is singular and blinding in the darkness. It is the light of the sun!

You pick up the pace once more and charge into the light of day. You see around you that you are in a slightly sparser area of the forest. Trees dot the area around you, but mostly it is a rocky terrain. You also see that you are much higher up than you were before. You can see another river many hundreds of feet below you. The trail continues ahead. You can see more than a mile of it, now that there are fewer trees to obstruct your view.

And off in the distance, to your surprise, you see

the Shadow! It is still running, faster than ever, along the trail. You catch a glimpse of it just before it disappears over a small hill.

You race to catch up to the Shadow, and hopeful thoughts rush through your mind. Maybe you had everything wrong. Maybe this creature is a captive of Brioxa as well. Maybe you two can help each other escape.

You are barely paying attention to your surroundings as you crest the hill that you saw the Shadow run over. As you charge up it, you look out to check for signs of the Shadow ahead of you. But instead, you find yourself staring out over a vast cliff.

And your momentum is carrying you over its edge.

Cliff

Your next step sends you flying off the edge of the cliff. You try to twist mid-air, desperate to grab at anything that can return you to solid ground. As gravity begins to take hold, you see a rush of green. Instinctively you reach out and grab hold of it, recognizing a sturdiness in your hands. You pull hard, and come to an abrupt halt in the air. Continuing to pull, you swing yourself back towards the face of the rock that makes up the cliff. You slam against the rock with a thud, then hang there for a moment, with your whole weight being supported by the branch or vine that you cling to. Scrambling up to the edge of the cliff, you pull yourself back onto horizontal ground.

You lay on your stomach, struggling to catch your breath for a moment. You take one deep breath.

In, holding for a moment, and then out.

Able to breath easily now, you stand up and approach the edge of the cliff again.

First, you notice the thing that saved you. It is a thick, green vine that stretches from the top of the cliff all the way to its bottom, which appears to be about 200 feet below. Then you take stock of the other features of the cliff. All along its sides, trees grow out at perfect 90-degree angles from the rock. These trees seem to be defying gravity completely. You look left and right along the edge of the cliff, and find that it extends for many miles, with no obvious way down to its bottom. The bottom of the cliff itself appears to be no different from the area that you have been walking through. There is a rocky area with a few trees, and a small path appearing to lead through it. In fact, as you peer down to the cliff's base, you can see what appears to be the path that you had been following, continuing directly below you.

You are astonished. Could this have been one continuous path once, before powerful forces deep within the earth chose to separate it? Is it expected that you would be able to make it down to the bottom of the cliff to pick up the trail once more?

You sit back and look around, examining the area on the edge of the cliff. Again, you see no easy way down. But off in the distance, a forest extends all the way to the horizon. Could the Shadow be out there somewhere?

You can just barely see some sort of structure rising up above the trees. It is many miles away, but it looks like it could be a village of some sort. Or perhaps you are just seeing what you want to see.

One thing is clear: there appear to be no other options. You need to climb down to the bottom of the cliff and take up the path again.

First you go to inspect the vine that you used to

save yourself just a few moments ago. Its origin is at the trunk of a tree that is no less than a few hundred years old. You yank on the vine once or twice to convince yourself that it will hold your weight. The vine holds firm, and puts your mind slightly more at ease.

You begin your descent by first wrapping the vine around your waste, and then slowly sliding off the edge of the cliff. Once you reach a few feet down, you move your feet so that your soles are flush against the rock. The vine is now pressed up against your lower back, and you are standing as if the face of the rock were flat ground. The slack of the vine is in your one hand, while the taught end leading back up to the sturdy tree is in the other. Carefully, you let out some of the slack and take a small step backwards. You let out just enough slack to match the step you take, and find yourself standing in the exact same position, but a foot lower on the face of the cliff.

You gradually increase your pace until the vine is constantly sliding through your hands at a slow speed. You are shocked at how light you feel. You had expected your descent to be more difficult. You are now walking backwards down the sheer cliff face at an almost casual pace.

Stopping briefly to check your surroundings, you are surprised to find that you are almost half-way down the cliff. Looking backwards towards the base of the wall, you see that your path is unobstructed by any of the trees that protrude from the rock face. You look back up at where you came from, and see some amount of movement.

The Shadow is standing at the edge of the cliff, right where you began your descent.

At first you remain still and hope that it does not see you, but that thought is quickly erased as it appears to lean down and peer at you. Perhaps it plans to follow you, in a role-reversal of sorts. For a time the Shadow stands, unmoving.

Just as you begin to debate calling out and trying to speak to it once more, you feel yourself drop slightly. The vine is giving way. You look around frantically to find some other rock or root to grab onto, but find nothing. You turn to your last hope: The Shadow. It could grab the vine and pull you back to the top.

"Help! The vine!", you shout, your free arm flailing for a moment before returning its grip to the vine. "I need you to pull me up!"

Then you hear that buzzing coming from the Shadow and see the true cause of your peril. Even from this distance you can see something in its hand. A rock, being swung at the vine. The creature must be trying to cut the vine and send you to your death!

"Stop, please! I haven't done anything to you!"

But your cries only serve to echo in the air as the vine finally gives way.

Your heart drops. Immediately you let go and begin to grasp around as gravity takes you once more. But this is a useless attempt. You know that there is nothing between your body and the hard ground 100 feet below. A wail escapes your mouth, as if a scream could slow your descent. Your eyes close, but no montage of your life passes before them. You see only blackness.

You feel a pressure under your armpits, and lurch to a stop mid-air. You find yourself continuing to scream, though danger has passed for the moment. Your eyes shoot open urgently, and you are desperate to find what force intervened. You are blinded by a brilliant light.

Brioxa.

You are not sure whether she dims herself or if your eyes adjust to her, but in any event, you find that you are now able to clearly see the Glowing Woman.

Her face shows no amusement as she holds you up. Her brow is furrowed, and her mouth forms a thin line. You look down to see that she is hovering in the air, supporting your weight as well. This new ability on her part does little to surprise you, however, given your experiences thus far. You look back to meet the gaze of her purple eyes.

"I am sorry." Brioxa says softly, but with a seriousness to her tone. "I was not expecting such resistance from it."

"Well, I'd say you made up for that." You gesture toward the ground. "Thanks."

Brioxa breaks her stare and avoids eye contact.

"I would not be so grateful."

Brioxa takes a step to her right and walks along the air as though there is a pane of glass beneath her feet. She still holds you very firmly beneath your armpits.

You feel like a toddler, and briefly debate struggling from her grip. You give up this thought when you look down again.

Brioxa is walking toward one of the trees jutting out from the side of the cliff. She turns and places you so that your legs straddle its horizontal trunk and lets go suddenly. Instinctively you reach down to grab hold of the branches of the tree and find that it is solid enough to hold your weight.

You let out a deep sigh. Brioxa is still staring at you with her eyebrows furrowed, creating creases in the golden skin of her forehead. The signs of concern are visible even in her strange features.

"What's wrong?", you venture to ask. Up to this point she has seemed all-knowing, and to see her so worried is deeply concerning.

"I am sad that I can help you no further." Again Brioxa looks away, ashamed.

You feel panic begin to creep up. You look around to see no other vines or holes in the rock to climb down. If she leaves, you will be stuck on the side of this cliff.

"Wait, but you can't just leave me here!"

But she is already retreating away.

"Stop!", you shout.

"I am sorry, but this journey is your own. Please know that I have the utmost faith in you." She smiles weakly and flies away, a streaking ray of light. She almost looks like a shooting star in the middle of the day.

You slam your fist into the trunk of the tree that you now sit on, but not too hard. You fear shaking its roots loose from the face of the cliff.

Looking left and right you again find nothing that you can grab hold of. Below you, though, is another tree just like the one you are sitting on, about ten feet down and slightly to your right. Maybe you could jump down, from tree to tree...

You shake your head and leave this thought. It would be far too dangerous.

Again you survey the surroundings, hoping for some beautifully easy solution to make itself obvious. And as you look around, you see a streak of black rush past you. The Shadow is falling towards the ground. You gasp and look on, horrified. Though it just tried to kill you, the thought of watching the creature's death does not excite you. As it reaches the ground, there is no loud thud or splat. The Shadow simply stops and tilts its head up at you, as if to brag of its ease in descending. Apparently feeling satisfied, it takes off up the trail once again, finally disappearing behind the trees.

You are offended by the smugness of the Shadow. You turn your attention much more seriously to the tree trunk a few feet below. There is another trunk a few feet below it, and another still below that one. You see now that you could leap between them and navigate your way to the base of the cliff.

You swing your left leg over the tree trunk that you have been sitting on, and eye the next trunk. Your legs dangle freely in the open air. You will need to gauge your leap very carefully, to avoid missing your mark and plummeting to your death. Something in Brioxa's tone makes you doubt that she will save you twice. You figure that you really will not need to jump, so much as fall to the next tree. It is almost perfectly below you.

You take a deep breathe, and slide off this tree and into a free fall. Air rushes mildly past your face as you drop. You tense all of your muscles, expecting to land hard on the trunk. You land with your stomach centered perfectly on the trunk of the tree, and scramble to grab a branch and steady yourself. But again, you find yourself much lighter than you would expect, and the landing is soft. Even the hard bark of the trunk did not seem to bring much pain as your stomach slammed into it. You lift yourself upright and catch your breath.

A smile crosses your face. Despite the stakes, that was fun.

You turn to see the next tree in your path. This one is slightly further down, and much further to your left. You bring your legs up and press the soles of your feet against the trunk of this tree. After steadying yourself, you push off and reach for the next tree.

This time, you reach out at grab a thick branch of the tree. You swing back and forth on the branch, trying to gain a hold of your balance as a gymnast might. When your swinging stops, you bring yourself up onto the trunk of the tree and find again that you enjoyed the trip. The whole process feels like very controlled flight.

You repeat this process over and over until you reach the base of the cliff. You drop the last few feet to the ground sadly, as you honestly enjoyed the climb.

Well, the parts that you were not plummeting to your death, anyway.

But the moment your feet touch solid ground you focus on the mission at hand. You must find the Shadow.

Cave

You begin to travel along the well-worn path again, choosing to walk rather than run. You fear moving too quickly and missing something important.

Like a cliff.

This section of the forest appears to be the same as the one you travelled through before the cliff, only with a bit more foliage. As you walk, you can clearly see through the branches overhead to the blue sky above. The surrounding brush is much less dark, making your task of looking for the Shadow simpler.

But you do not see it. After a long effort of searching carefully along the path, you find yourself falling back into the habit of admiring the surrounding plant life. Many colors attract your eye.

At one point, you stop to carefully inspect a little blue bush. Its leaves are long and come to a point, reminding you of a small palm tree. Under its shade, a small cloud of the glowing, bodiless bugs hovers. You take the time to inspect them again and still find that they have no substance, just a point of light floating in the air. You take one of the leaves of the bush and cup your hands around it. You peer into the dark space that you have created and find that the leaves glow, too. This whole area must be wonderful after the sun sets.

You continue to walk and find that the path is leading you into a rock outcropping surrounded by dense forest. This must be the structure that you saw from the top of the cliff. In your obsession with the Shadow you had forgotten all about your desire to find civilization, and even now you hardly feel the weight of this disappointment. You can find your way home after you have confronted this beast.

You stand at the base of the rock and look up, debating the merits of climbing to the top. Maybe from such a height you could see the Shadow.

Just then, as if in answer to your thought, you see some movement near a boulder to your left. You hurry to inspect the area and find a cave in the side of the rock. You strain your eyes against the darkness of the cave, and again see some sort of motion within the shadows. You cannot be sure, yet you believe the Shadow must be in there. But is it wise to approach it in the darkness, where it will have the advantage?

You take a deep breath. In, and out.

You must dive in. If the Shadow is in there, it will be cornered and forced to face you. Perhaps you two might even be able to come to an understanding, and help each other overtake Brioxa and escape this place.

Yet you do not feel very confident in this last idea. You lean down and pick up a rock, about the size of your fist. If the Shadow attacks again, you will be ready.

You step into the cave, finding its uneven floor somewhat difficult to walk on. After a few steps you cannot see. You wish those glowing plants grew here, too. Then it dawns on you: the matches from the windmill!

In your pocket you find the little box, and fumble in the dark to pull one out and strike it. Finally you are successful, and the whole area around you explodes with light.

The cave appears to be one large chamber with a rather low ceiling. All of the walls around you are jagged and uneven, matching the floor beneath your feet. The rock of the walls is a cool grey color, with veins of white streaking through. Across from you, there are a few openings in the rock wall. Five of them, in fact. The largest opening is on the left, with each getting progressively smaller to the right.

As you inspect these new tunnels, you notice something strange between them. The light from your match is hitting the area between the first and second tunnels strangely. As you move to look more closely, the flame of the match finally makes its way down to your fingers, burning them. You drop the match quickly and the light goes out.

You hurry to pull out another match and light it. As the light refills the cave, you find that now it is hitting much more of the wall strangely. Then suddenly there is movement. The Shadow stands right in front of you. It must have tried to approach you in the darkness. Now it seems to turn and retreat into one of the openings, the second from the left.

You chase after the Shadow, but do not call out. Speaking to it has not gotten you anywhere thus far, and you no longer believe it understands. You make your way through the opening and find a tunnel. The light fills this smaller space well, bouncing off all of the jagged walls. You run through, scanning around. You fear the Shadow slipping back out and know this may be your only chance to corner it.

After running for maybe a hundred feet, the tunnel comes to an abrupt halt. You can see an opening in the rock at its very end, with some amount of dim light shining through, but you do not focus on this for long. You must find the Shadow.

You wave the match around, spreading its light to find the creature, when you hear a high-pitched buzzing sound. You move towards the awful sound, and find that it only grows louder and more worried. Finally, in the furthest corner of this alcove, you find the Shadow.

You move the match so that it is between you and the Shadow, and cock back the rock in your hand, ready to strike. You see that the creature is curled up into a ball and shakes uncontrollably. The air seems to be rippling around it in response to the buzzing sound. The light hurts it, but you cannot afford to blind yourself for its comfort. Still, you feel confident enough in your position that you drop the rock. If need be, you will use the light to scare the Shadow away.

You kneel down in front of it, hoping to get a closer look. The buzzing lessens, and the Shadow seems to turn its head to inspect you. You put both hands out in front of you, hoping to show that you do not mean any harm. The Shadow flinches at first, as one of your hands still holds a match. But then the buzzing almost completely dies out.

The Shadow seems particularly interested in the light of the match, though it will not get too close. Carefully, you try to extend the match to it, so that it could look more closely. The Shadow flinches away again, but then it makes some sort of realization. It uncurls from its ball and appears to even relax. Maybe the light does not wound it after all.

Suddenly all around you is dark again, and you realize that the match must have once again gone out. You scramble to retrieve another match and light it. This may be your only chance to make peace with the Shadow, and you do not want to let it escape before you find common ground. You are finally able to strike another match, and then scan the cave frantically. But the Shadow has not moved since the last match went out. It still sits on the floor of the cave, its head tilted curiously towards you.

The Shadow's one hand reaches out, gently, towards the match. You hand it to the creature, and it brings the source of light gradually closer to its face. The Shadow seems mystified by the light. You watch it with great interest as the light does nothing to illuminate its features. The Shadow remains only that, a silhouette against the flicker of the match's light.

With its inspection of the match complete, the Shadow turns its attention back to you. Seeming much calmer now, it extends its hand towards you. You flinch suddenly, unsure if this is a sign of peace or something else, but the Shadow remains unmoved. You decide that this is your best chance to make a connection with this being, and return the gesture.

The moment your hands touch, the Shadow's appearance changes drastically. Its features are now clear in the dim light of the match.

And its face is your own.

You stare, shocked at this being, as if you were staring into a twisted mirror. Every feature on the face and body are exactly like that of your own, save for a few exceptions. Where eyes would be on your own face, there are only pits of the deepest darkness. The mouth hangs open lifelessly, and its hair is matted and mussed. Its skin is dark grey, and its cheeks are sunken. The whole thing is truly terrible to look at, and yet you cannot look away.

"What are you?", you manage to croak out through your surprise.

The Shadow's mouth curls into a gentle, knowing smile, and realization dawns on you.

Just then, the match finally burns out, and darkness surrounds you once more. In your shock, you do not even reach for another match. But the darkness does not last long. Soon a bright glow appears from behind you. It lights the cave just in time for you to see the Shadow fly through the tunnel and back out of the cave.

You turn around to face Brioxa. She smiles at you with pride in her eyes.

"I've been to this place before," you begin.

"Many times, yes," Brioxa responds gently. "In times of great distress, and otherwise."

"And that thing, it's..."

"A part of you, yes. You two have been through this struggle many times before. But it always ends the same."

You sit and think on these words. This all feels so familiar now. You look down at the cloak, still wrapped around your body, and see that the symbols make complete sense to you now. It is your name, written over and over in a hundred different ways, all of them in gold.

Without needing to ask what the next step is, you turn to the crack in the rock wall. It is just big enough that you could crawl through it. On the other side, you see the same misty nothingness that surrounded you when you first awoke on the side of the mountain, where you thought the Glowing Woman had left you to die.

"This is all your creation," she continues.

You turn back to face her and admire her glowing gold skin, and pupil-less purple eyes. They seem to you the most comforting sight in all of existence.

"You keep this place hidden within yourself, so that you might explore it when you have the need."

You think through this information, and it lights a realization in you.

Head.

Neck.

Chest.

Heart.

Back.

Stomach.

Thighs.

Knees.

Feet.

You have been travelling within yourself.

"And I put you here to help me?" The details are still foggy for you, but becoming ever clearer.

"Only when times are truly dire," she says with a smile. "It was very important to you that this journey be yours and yours alone. Often times you pass through without any need of me at all."

Suddenly you become concerned of the Shadow's presence in this world of your own creation.

"That... thing... will it continue to haunt this place forever?"

"I suspect so, yes," Brioxa says with a thoughtful nod. "But each time you two interact I notice a change in it, and in you. To me, you both seem more at peace with one another. It seems almost as if you are both wearing away at each other."

With this sentence her purple eyes softened, and Brioxa seems to look on at you with genuine affection.

You turn back to the crack in the wall.

"And this will lead me back out into the world, right? The real world?" You are not able to hide the disappointment in your voice as you consider abandoning these realizations that you have fought so hard to reach.

"Yes, it will."

"And have I ever just stayed in this place?"

"For a time, yes," Brioxa says after a moment. "But eventually you always choose to walk out, holding onto what you have learned here."

You whirl to face her.

"And what have I learned here?"

She laughs sweetly at the question, like an adult might at a child who asks if heaven is real.

"Well, it is something new every time, really. That is why you come back."

You ponder this for a moment. What is it that you have learned here? What new lesson is there?

Brioxa seems curious of your decision as well, and stares at you with the faintest remains of a smile still lingering on her face. You stand up and turn to the portal. You step towards it.

This whole time you have been in a realm of your own creation, a world that seems so untamable though it resides within you. As with all things, there are foreboding shadows and imperfections. But there is beauty here as well, and no one is more responsible for this beauty than you. While the dark pits in your own mind may never leave you, the brilliance will not either.

You must hold onto that notion as you make your way through the real world, where things are no less mysterious and confusing. And you must come back here, you think. Something deep within you knows that, if left unchecked, this world and all of its wonders will crumble.

Who knows, maybe you will even be able to work hand-in-hand with that Shadow one day. A partnership between you could bring great things for this world, and for you both.

Just before you step toward the opening, you feel arms wrap around you. Brioxa squeezes you with a hug. Her light seems to warm you to your core and fill you with hope. A tear of happiness rolls down your cheek.

"I love you, and you created me," she says softly. "So, please, love yourself."

Brioxa lets you go, and you begin to crawl through the crevasse, and back into the murky grey. You will be back in your room and in your bed soon.

"Good luck!" Brioxa beckons after you, just before you reach the end of the passage.

And so, you step forward, armed with the knowledge that if you can make peace with the dark recesses of your mind, then the real world will be a walk in the park.

About the Author and Artist

John O'Neill is an author currently living in Columbus, OH. He is a graduate of The Ohio State University, whose day job is designing roads as a civil engineer. His hobbies include reading comic books, camping, and sleeping through his alarm.

Jayne Kennedy is a fine artist based in Cincinnati, OH. She is currently interested in painting vibrant, cloud-centric imagery. In her free time, she enjoys a good nature hike or a fun video game (preferably an RPG). Her work can be viewed both on her website www.artofjayne.com, and on her Instagram @artofjayne.

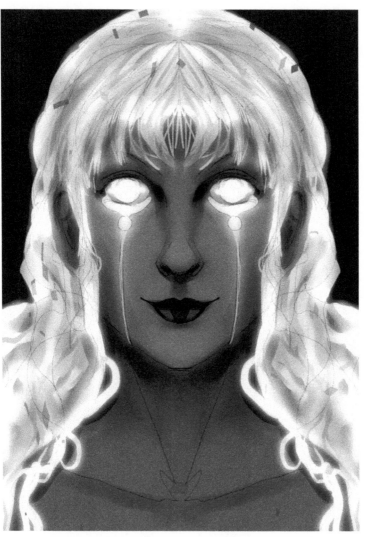

"In my brain, she's hot ... and kinda scary."
Jayne on Brioxa

Aknowledgements

This book is the result of endless encouragement and critiques from the people that I love. I need to thank Brandon and Ray for reading through this and giving me sincere feedback. Of course thanks to Brian, who asked for the manuscript, even if he never opened it. And finally Colin, who egged me on and told me he would only read it after it had been published. There were so many people who influenced this story over the years it took me to finish it, and I hope they all know that it was appreciated in a way that exceeds just words.